Understanding Body, Breath & Balance

YOGA FOR KIDS

Bhushan Patwardhan
Eeha Kulkarni

With

Arjun Hingorani and Sariva Tillu

Designed by

Pallavi Vywahare

Domain Knowledge Associate

Kaivalyadhama, Lonavala

Sakāl
Publications

Sakal Publications

YOGA FOR KIDS

Sakal Media Pvt. Ltd.
595, Budhwar Peth,
Pune—411002, India

www.sakalpublications.com
sakalprakashan@esakal.com

First Edition: December 2025

ISBN No.: 978-93-89834-96-3

Designed by: Pallavi Vyawahare

Printed in India by Sakal Media Pvt. Ltd.

Before This book is Dedicated To We Begin

Rayakaka Patwardhan, who may not have practiced Yoga in form but lived its essence through sports, simplicity, compassion, and balance.

And

Ramkumar Rathi, a visionary entrepreneur and philanthropist whose life was devoted to serving humanity and sharing the light of Yoga.

Their lives reflected a deep spiritual awareness and the true spirit of Yoga — gentle, aware, and deeply humane.

About This Book

Yoga for Kids isn't just another history, fiction, or exercise book. It's a curious, creative guide to help you grow smart, kind, and strong from the inside out. Join Ravi, Tara, and their wise friend Uncle Vivek as they explore:

- Stories of Yoga-loving icons from sports, music, and movies
- Simple stretches and breathing tricks for energy and focus
- Daily habits to feel better at school, in sports, and at home
- Fun games, journal prompts, and experiments
- Ancient secrets made playful for today's kids

A Promise

No pressure. No preaching. Just tools for the most important journey of all—exploring yourself. Whether you love football or books, dancing or doodling, this book shows how Yoga meets you where you are, and helps you shine.

So... let your adventure begin!

Disclaimer

This book introduces Yoga as a knowledge system for children in simple and engaging terms. Stories and examples are used to explain complex ideas, though they may not always capture their full classical depth. The aim is to spark curiosity and present Yoga in an educative, interesting, and thoughtful way while staying true to its core philosophy.This is not a practice manual. Children should not attempt any Yoga postures or techniques on their own. Yoga must always be learned under the guidance of a qualified teacher and with the supervision of parents or guardians. The pictures in this book are only basic illustrations to show the idea of a pose, not exact versions to follow. Yoga is a vast subject with advanced practices like *nāḍī* systems, *śuddhikriyā*, and various *mudras*, which are not covered here; as children grow, they can learn these in detail from trained teachers.

Content Guide

"Yoga has a complete message for humanity."
- Swami Kuvalayananda, Founder, Kaivalyadhama

Part IV - Balance & Science

Part V - Adventure & Beyond

Annexures

Foreword

"Each soul is potentially divine. The goal is to manifest this divinity within."
- Swami Vivekananda

Yoga for Kids: Understanding Body, Breath & Balance introduces Yoga as one of the most precious knowledge traditions of Bharat. It is a timeless way of living that helps us stay healthy in body, peaceful in mind, and kind in heart. This is not a book that teaches how to do Yoga, but one that helps readers understand it as a way of life that builds awareness, balance, and inner strength.

For many years, I have written hundreds of research papers and scholarly books meant for grown-ups. Yet, in the changing times we live in, I feel it is even more important to help young minds appreciate our rich knowledge heritage. That thought led to the creation of Ayurveda for Kids, and now Yoga for Kids continues that journey. Children need to understand the value of India's knowledge systems from an early age. The National Education Policy (NEP) 2020 also encourages schools to include Indian Knowledge Systems in their curriculum. This book supports that vision by introducing Yoga in a simple, enjoyable, and thoughtful way that young readers can relate to.

My own journey with Yoga began at home, inspired by my parents. I was fortunate to learn from many great teachers who introduced me to the science of Yoga, including Drs. M. V. Bhole, M. L. Gharote, and M. V. Rajapurkar at Kaivalyadhama, founded by Swami Kuvalayananda. Later, my interactions with Drs. O. P. Tiwari, Samprasad Vinod, Vishwas Mandlik, B. N. Gangadhar, H. R. Nagendra, Nagarathna, Sri Sri Ravi Shankar, Swami Ramdeo, Gururaj Mutalik, and many others deepened my understanding. They helped me see that Yoga is not only about postures or breathing, but about living with awareness, compassion, and harmony.

I am delighted that Kaivalyadhama, now celebrating its centenary, has joined us as our Domain Knowledge Associate. As Chair of its Research Advisory Committee, I hold deep respect for this pioneering institution that bridges the wisdom of Yoga and the rigor of science. I am also grateful to its CEO, Shri Subodh Tiwari, with whom I share a long and valued friendship.

Today, children grow up surrounded by screens, distractions, and endless information. Yoga for Kids hopes to bring them moments of calm and reflection. Through simple stories, examples, and activities, it invites both children and adults to explore how Yoga can bring peace, kindness, and confidence into everyday life. May this book inspire every reader to pause, breathe, and discover the joy of balance — within and around them.

Dr. Bhushan Patwardhan, PhD, FNASc, FAMS
Former Vice Chairman University Grants Commission
National Research Professor-Ayush
Ramkumar Rathi Patanjali Yoga Chair
Interdisciplinary School of Health Sciences
Savitribai Phule Pune University
Pune, India

Before We Begin

"The art of staying calm and balanced in all situations is true Yoga."
समत्वं योग उच्यते – Bhagavad Gita 2.48

Modern life is fast-paced. Kids grow up with TikTok, Roblox, Netflix, and endless notifications. Many are pressurized to score well, shine in sports, keep up with friends, and meet family expectations. It is exciting—but also stressful.

This book is your companion on this journey! It introduces Yoga not as something old or boring, but as a practical way to feel stronger, calmer, and more alive.

Meet Your Friends!

- **Tara** - A cheerful and compassionate girl who once felt tired from schoolwork and too much screen time, until she discovered how Yoga could lift her mood and brighten her day. (Tara means "Star" — a symbol of hope.)
- **Ravi** - Tara's curious younger brother, full of questions and energy, always eager to explore and learn. (Ravi means "Sun" — a symbol of energy and light.)
- **Uncle Vivek** - A wise family friend and scientist who loves connecting ancient wisdom with modern science. (Vivek means "Wisdom.")

Together, they will journey through Yoga, guided by curiosity — asking, testing, and playing as they go.

Yoga Is Everywhere

Look closely, you'll notice Yoga already around you: Cristiano Ronaldo and Virat Kohli use Yoga for focus and flexibility. Steve Jobs used to meditate, Lady Gaga and Oprah practice it to handle stress. Members of

K-pop groups BTS and BLACKPINK meditate to stay calm. Even Kung Fu Panda's Po learns inner peace!

And Roald Dahl (Matilda) said, "Those who don't believe in magic will never find it." And Mufasa (The Lion King, Disney) said, "Look inside yourself, Simba. You are more than what you have become."

That's what Yoga teaches: Your amazing superpowers are already within!

A Story That Began Long Ago

Legends say Yoga began with Shiva, the first yogi. Later, Patanjali organized Yogic teachings into the Yoga Sutras, a guide to values, breath, postures, and meditation. From forests and mountains, Yoga travelled across cultures and continues to evolve today.

Science Catches Up

What sages practiced long ago is now proven by science:

- Brain scans show Yoga improves memory and focus.
- Studies show it reduces stress, improves sleep, and helps kids with ADHD.
- Even NASA uses breathing techniques for astronauts in space.

How to Use This Book

This isn't a rulebook. It is a friendly adventure with stories, science, and simple practices. Look for:

- "Try This!" boxes - small experiments and games
- Notes to Self - Ravi & Tara's doodles and reflections
- Fun facts + Science connections

You don't need to believe everything. Just stay curious, try little things, and notice what happens.

What's Inside

• Part I: Why Yoga matters today, plus stories and symbols

• Part II: Meet your amazing body and learn strong poses

• Part III: Discover your breath and mind power

• Part IV: Explore deeper maps—layers, energies, chakras, science

• Part V: Bring Yoga into daily life—routines, tech balance, games, and safety

• Glossary + Surya Namaskar guide at the end.

We firmly believe that the Bhagavad Gita states, "Yoga is the journey of the self, through the self, to the self". Bangtan Boys - K- Pop Band, BTS

Part I

Introduction & Inspiration

"It's not about how much you have. It's about how much you enjoy."
- Po, Kung Fu Panda

Why Yoga still matters in a busy, digital world? Before poses and breathwork, let's pause and ask:

- Why do kids today feel so rushed and distracted?
- Can an ancient practice really help with school, screens, and stress?
- What stories and symbols keep Yoga alive even today?

This part invites you to be curious. Meet Ravi, Tara, and Uncle Vivek as they explore everyday life, big questions, and the ancient stories of Yoga.

1. Hello, Yoga Buddies!

"Adventure is out there!"
- Up (Pixar)

A soft morning glow filled the family room as Ravi bounced onto his mat and Tara rolled hers out beside him. Their Uncle Vivek, both guide and scientist, settled between them with a warm smile.

Ravi hopped forward. "Uncle Vivek, I feel awake this morning... but how can Yoga make my energy last all day?"

Tara stretched her arms overhead. "I need to focus on my school project. Can Yoga help me too?"

Uncle Vivek nodded. "Great questions! Think of it as a tune-up for your body, a refresh button for your mind, and a steady rhythm for your breath. Yoga is not about fancy tricks or competition."

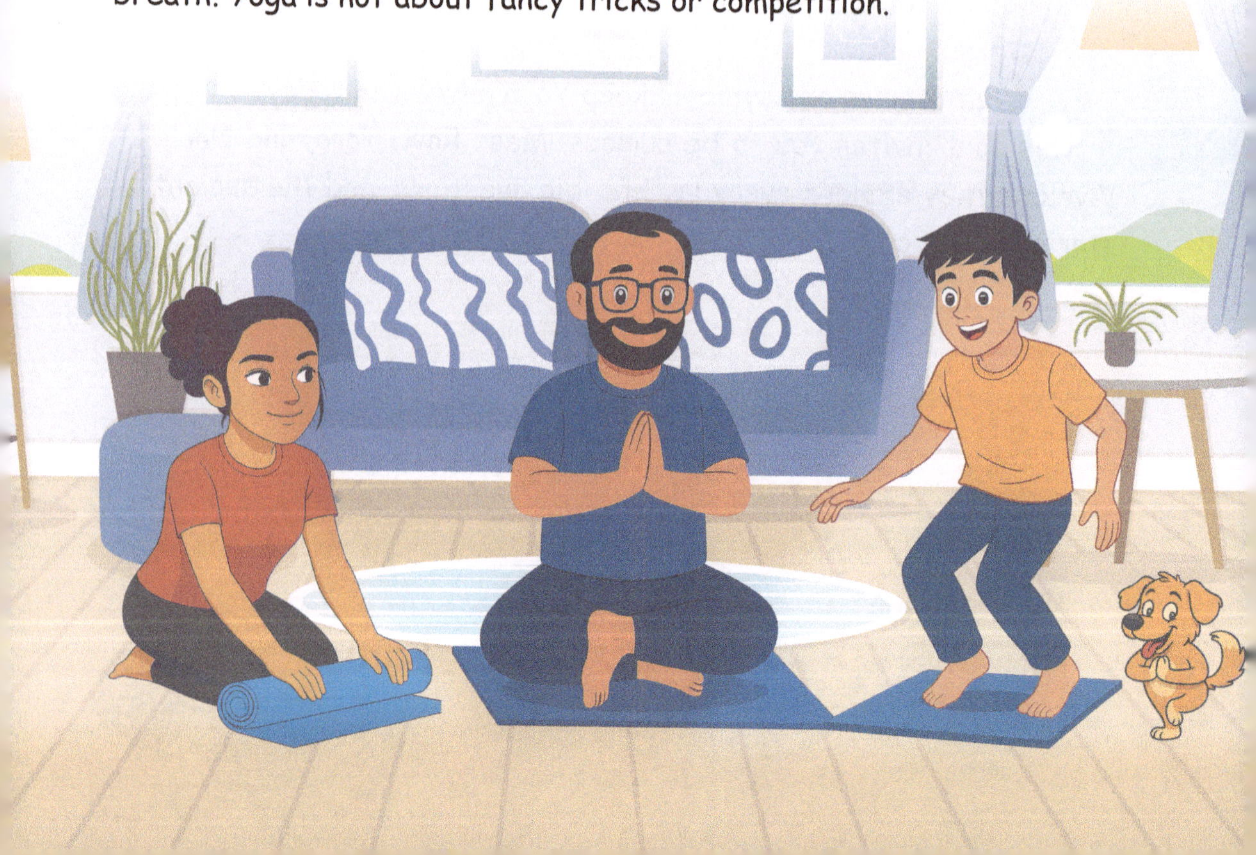

What Do You Think Yoga Is?

Uncle Vivek asked, "When you hear the word Yoga, what do you picture?"

"Touching toes," Ravi said.

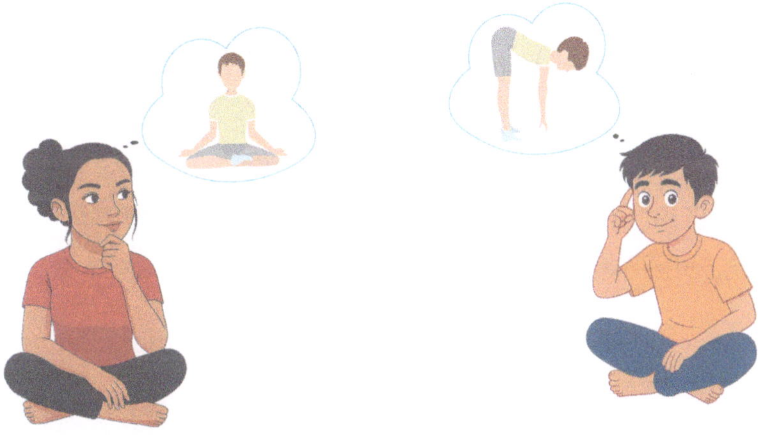

"Sitting cross-legged and saying Om," Tara added. "Animal poses—like Cobra and Dog!" Ravi grinned.

"Sure," Uncle Vivek nodded. "Those are parts of Yoga. But Yoga is much more. It's about understanding and balancing yourself."

What Is Yoga?

The word Yoga comes from the Sanskrit yuj, which has many meanings, and one of them is "to join" or "to unite." Each time you practice, you join body, breath, and mind—or even connect yourself with the bigger universe.

Yoga's Three Gifts

* **Focus** - Watching your breath helps your mind concentrate, perfect for schoolwork or tests.
* **Calm** - Gentle movements and steady breathing relax your body after stress or screen time.
* **Strength** - Holding postures like Warrior or Tree builds steady muscles and balance.

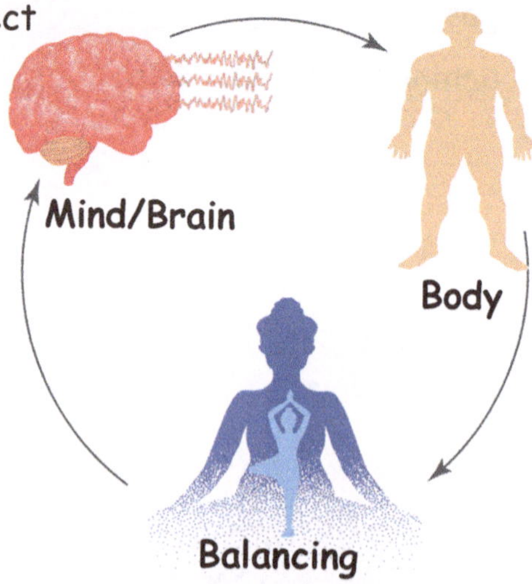

Yoga in Action

Ravi wobbled in Tree Pose with his eyes gazed at one point. "Whoa! This is harder than it looks!"

Uncle Vivek smiled. "See? Yoga isn't about touching the ground—it's about finding balance inside and out."

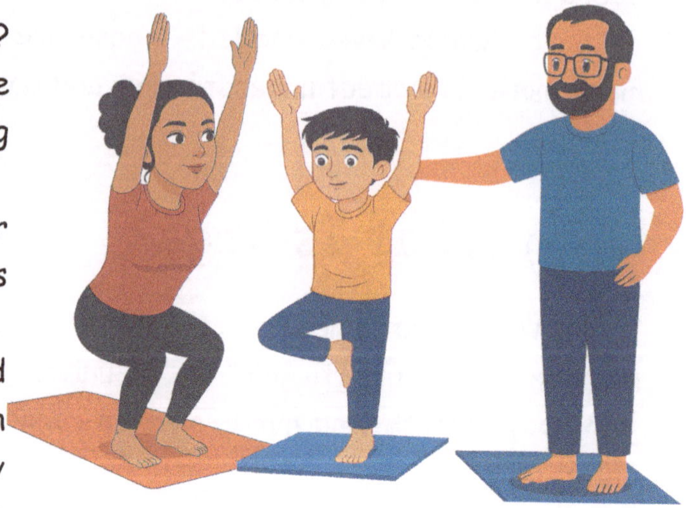

Tara crouched into Chair Pose. "And what about poses you hold for a long time?"

"That's where strength and discipline comes in. You learn to breathe steadily and stay present—qualities that help in exams, sports, and even family challenges."

Try This!

Simple Breath Tune-Up

1. Sit tall with a straight spine.
2. Inhale through your nose for 4 counts.
3. Exhale through your nose for 4 counts.
4. Repeat 5 times.

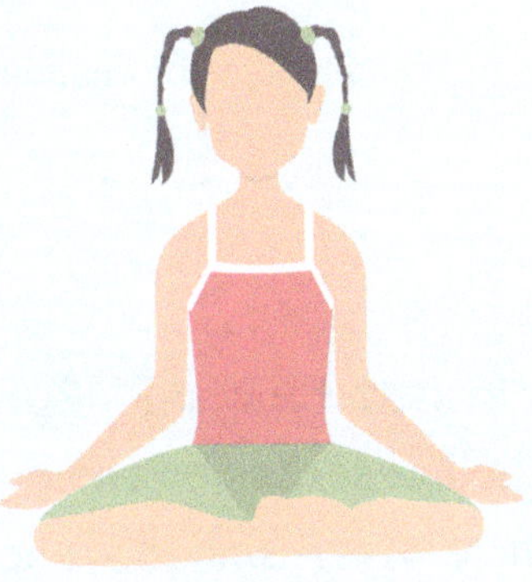

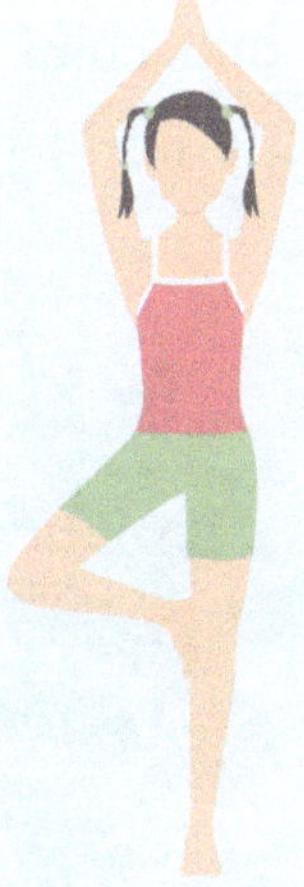

Mini Tree Pose

1. Stand with feet hip-width apart.
2. Shift weight onto one foot; place the other on calf or ankle (not on the knee).
3. Hands at heart or reaching up like branches.
4. Hold for 10 seconds, then switch sides.

Takeaway

» Yoga connects your body, breath, and thoughts into one team.

» It gives 3 gifts: focus, calm, and strength.

» Poses are not tricks; they're tools for balance in daily life.

2. Can Yoga Really Help? - The Case for Curiosity

"It is not our abilities that show what we truly are... it is our choices."
- Dumbledore, Harry Potter

Ravi leaned forward. "But how can stretching or breathing really fix things like stress or tiredness?"

Uncle Vivek smiled. "Yoga doesn't 'fix' you like a mechanic fixes a car. It teaches you how your body, breath, and mind work together. Once you understand, small changes ripple everywhere."

He drew a scribble on one page of his notebook and calm waves on another. "This is your mind on a stressful day... and this is your mind after steady breathing."

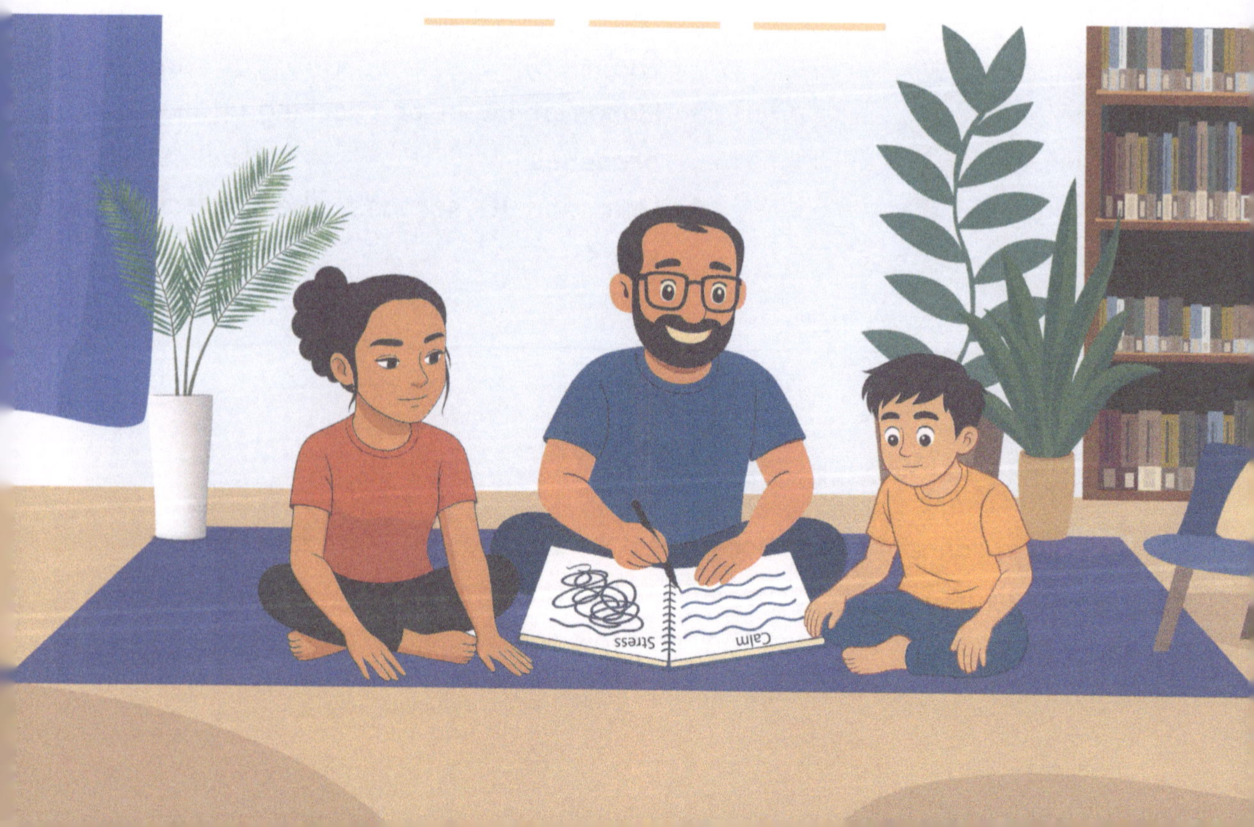

Ancient but Not Outdated

Tara frowned. "But isn't Yoga... old? Is it really that important nowadays?"

"Yes, Yoga is ancient," Uncle Vivek replied. "But modern science is catching up."

- Brain scans show Yoga increases memory and focus areas.
- Studies reveal Yoga helps sleep and reduces anxiety.
- What sages explored in forests, scientists now measure in labs.

"Whoa," Ravi whispered. "So, Yoga is like a science experiment on myself?"

"Exactly," Uncle Vivek nodded. "A living science you can test and trust."

Curiosity Is the Key

"You don't need to believe everything I say", Uncle Vivek said. "The only requirement for Yoga is curiosity and persistence."

Tara nodded. "That's what happened to me. The first time I noticed my breath calming me down, I knew it worked!"

Ravi grinned. "So, Yoga isn't about touching toes—it's about touching curiosity?"

The Power of Breath

Uncle Vivek placed one hand on his chest and one on his belly.

"When you guide your breath—what Yoga calls pranayama—you send more oxygen to your brain and muscles. A few deep breaths can calm you before a test or freshen you up when you are tired."

Ravi inhaled deeply. "It's like charging my batteries!"

Tara closed her eyes. "When I focus on my breath, my thoughts stop jumping."

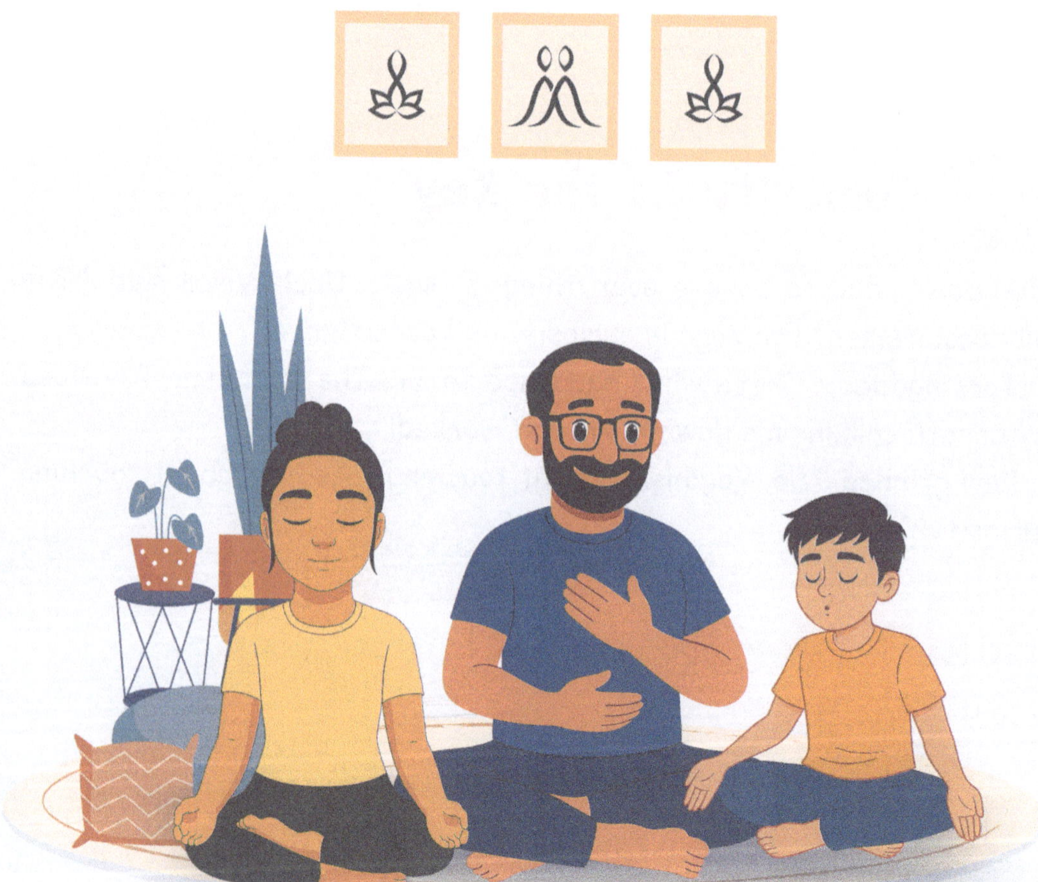

Try This!

Curiosity Test

Before practice, ask:

- What do I notice in my body?
- How does my breath feel—fast, slow, shallow, deep?
- What changes after one minute of practice?

Draw or write your answers. Nothing is right or wrong!

Balance & Focus

1. Stand in Tree Pose.
2. Close eyes. Feel tiny body adjustments.
3. Breathe for 5 counts.

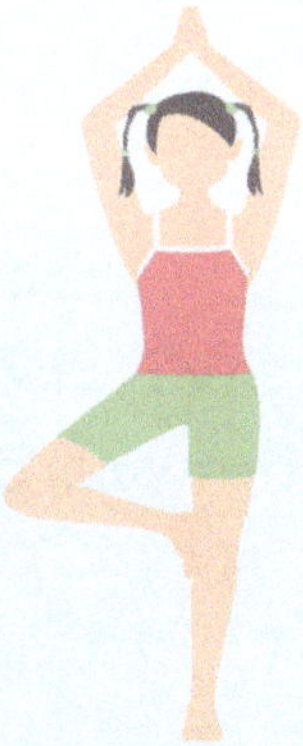

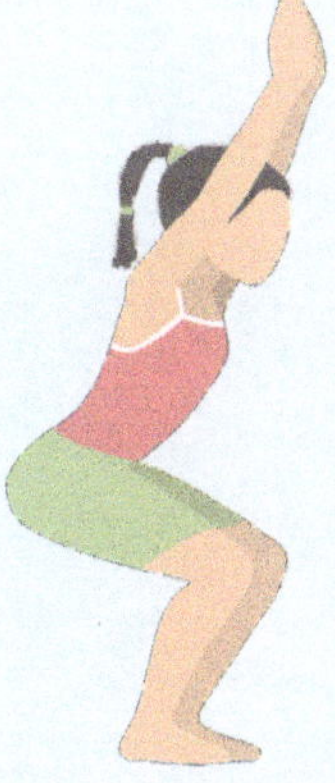

Strength & Breath

1. Hold Chair Pose.
2. Inhale for 4 counts, exhale for 4.
3. Stay for 5 breaths.

Mindful Moment

1. Sit comfortably, hand on heart.
2. Take 5 slow breaths.
3. Notice how your mind feels after.

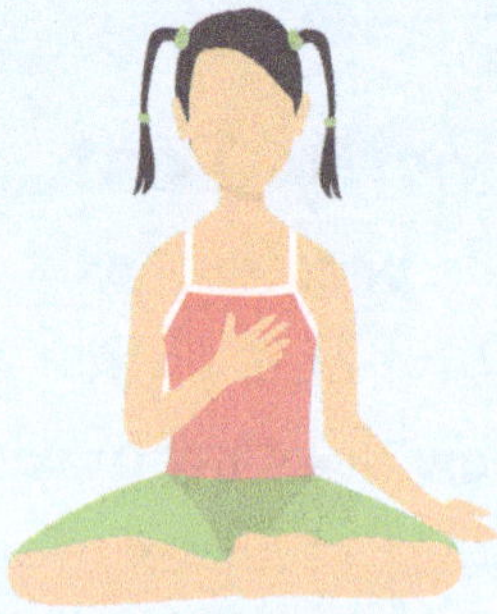

TAKEAWAY

- Yoga is not about tricks, it's a living science.
- Curiosity is the only entry ticket.
- Breath = your battery charger for body and mind.

3. Growing Up in a Busy World

"Slow down and enjoy life. It's not only the scenery you miss by going too fast, you also miss the sense of where you are going."
- The Tortoise and the Hare

Tara looked out the window. Traffic buzzed, phones pinged, screens glowed. Ravi sat in pajamas juggling three devices at once—tablet, phone, and TV.

"Do you even know what you're watching?" Tara teased.

"Kind of," Ravi grinned. "A game walkthrough, an animal reel, and... some math video that started by accident."

Tara laughed, but she remembered when her brain also felt like a browser with too many tabs open.

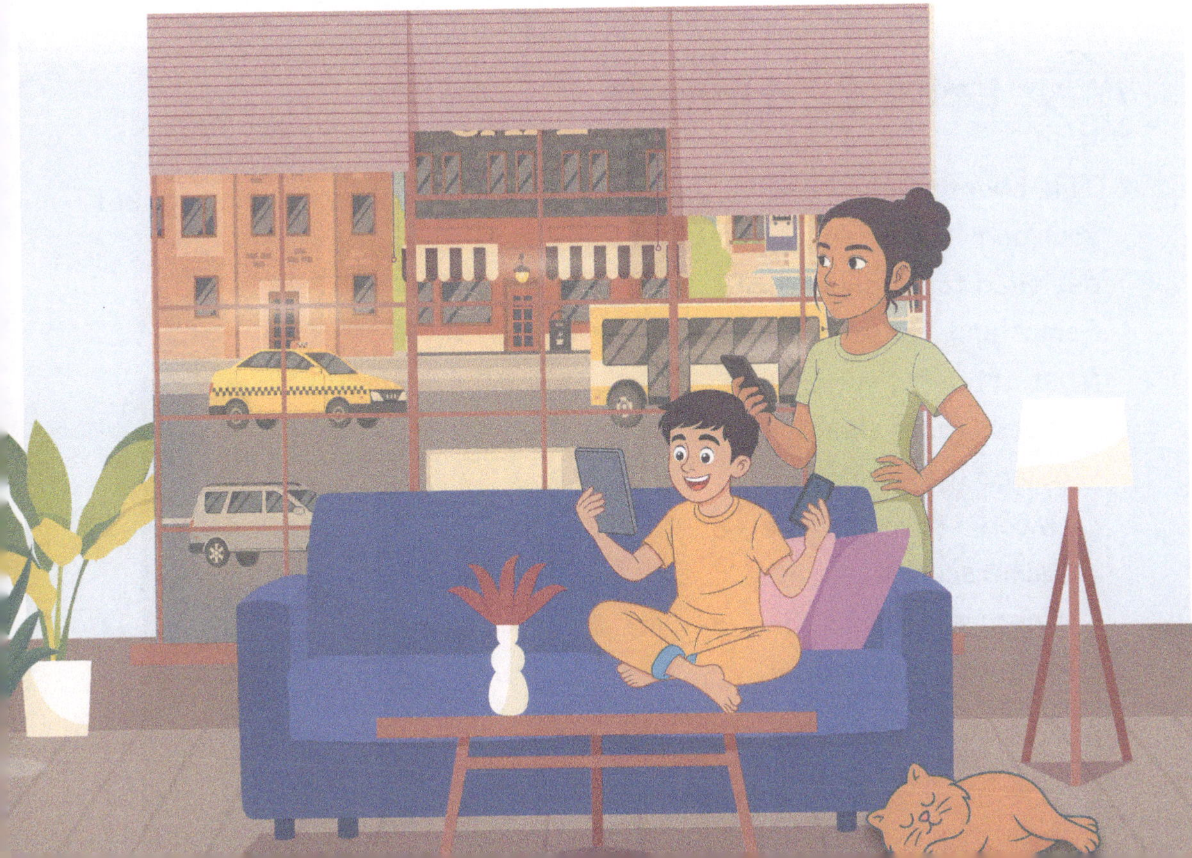

Welcome to the "Always On" World

Kids today juggle schoolwork, notifications, sports, hobbies, and family expectations. Everyone says "do your best," but no one explains what to do when "best" feels like it's not enough.

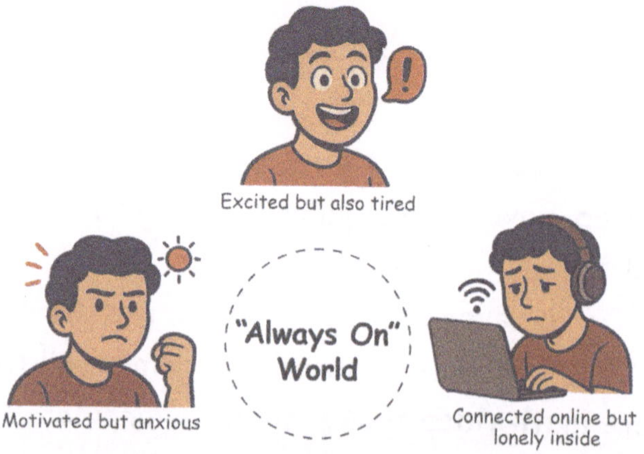

Sometimes you might feel:

- Excited but also tired
- Connected online but lonely inside
- Motivated but anxious

That's not just you—that's the world around you.

Let's Be Honest

This chapter isn't here to blame screens. Technology is amazing. But your body and brain weren't designed for endless speed. Something has to give. Most often it's your:

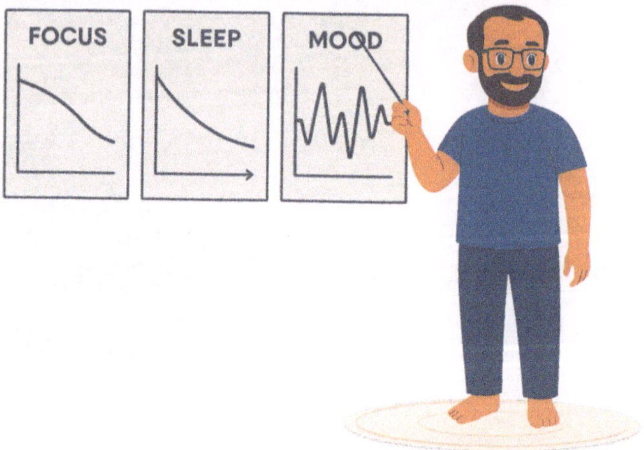

- Focus (gets shorter)
- Sleep (gets delayed)
- Mood (swings like a game score)
- Posture (slumps like a melted marshmallow)

Your Body Is Always Listening

One evening, Ravi lost a game and slammed his controller. His shoulders tightened, breath went fast, and his stomach churned.

"Relax," Tara said, handing him water.

Uncle Vivek explained: "Your body is always listening to your thoughts, emotions, and breath. When life feels overwhelming, your body shows it."

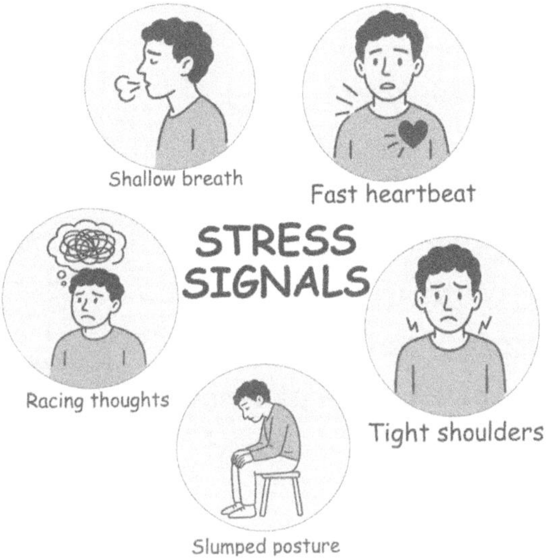

Stress signals include:

- Shallow breath
- Fast heartbeat
- Tight shoulders
- Slumped posture
- Racing thoughts

The Science of Stress

"Your brain has an alarm system," Uncle Vivek said. "It releases hormones like adrenaline when you're scared or pressured. Long ago, that helped humans run from tigers. Today, the same alarm goes off for tests, deadlines, or rejection."

"That's why we need better tools," Tara said. "Not ignoring stress, but calming it."

Your Brain: A Brilliant Machine

Your brain needs fuel beyond food:

- Good sleep
- Movement
- Focused attention
- Quiet time
- Healthy breathing

Without these, kids often feel tired or anxious. That's not laziness—it's overload

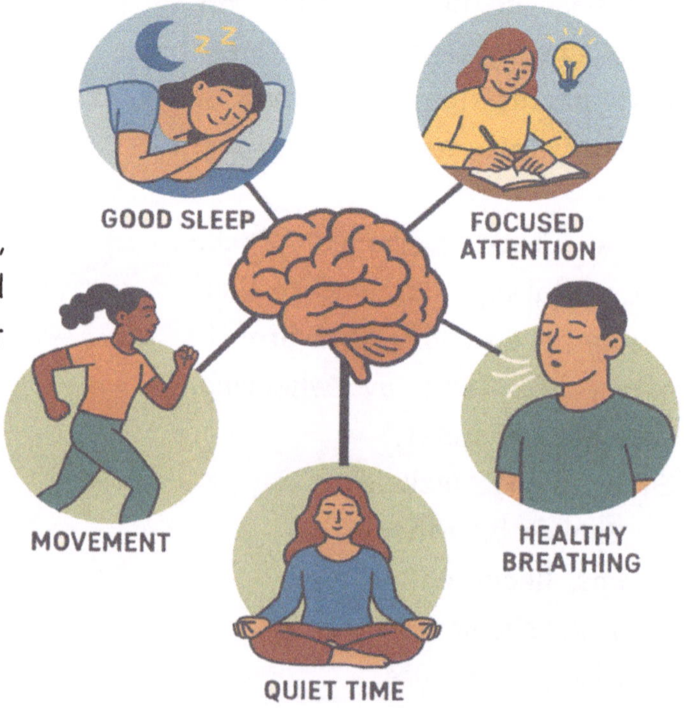

The Body-Mind Connection

"Your body and mind are a team," Uncle Vivek said.

- Tension in body — racing thoughts.
- Racing thoughts — more tension in body.
- Bad breathing makes it worse.
- Good movement and mindful breath flip the switch.

You're Not Alone

Kids everywhere—from New York to Nairobi to Mumbai—face the same pressures. Many are clever and creative, but also exhausted.

"That's how this book guides you," Uncle Vivek said. "Not to make you perfect yogis, but to make your life happy and positive: with strength, awareness, calm, and clarity."

Tara smiled.

Ravi still loved the internet, but both were learning that slowing down could actually help them go faster in the right way.

Try This!

Simple Breath Tune-Up

1. Sit with a straight back.
2. Inhale slowly from your belly.
3. Exhale slowly and completely.
4. Repeat 5 times.
5. Notice how your jaw and thoughts soften.

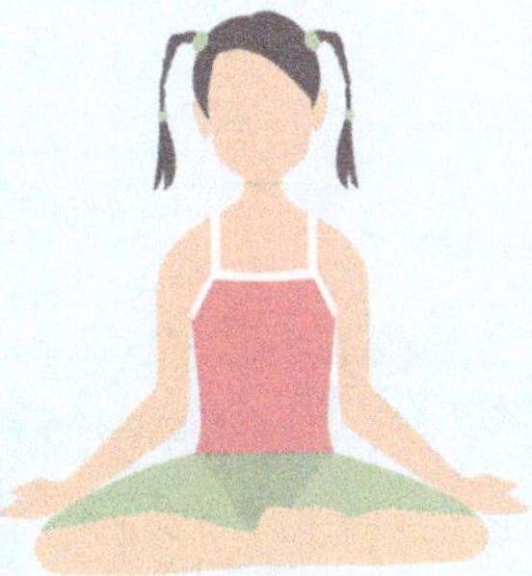

TAKEAWAY

- The "always on" world is exciting but tiring.
- Stress shows in your body and mind.
- Your breath and awareness are the best reset tools.
- Slowing down sometimes makes life smoother.

4. The Story and Symbols of Yoga

"The past can hurt. But the way I see it, you can either run from it or learn from it."
- Rafiki, The Lion King

Ravi and Tara perched on their yoga mats and exchanged quick glances, both wondering if yoga would be as exciting as the stories said.

"Uncle Vivek," Ravi asked, "was Yoga invented yesterday?" Tara giggled. "I heard it's very old. What's the real story?"

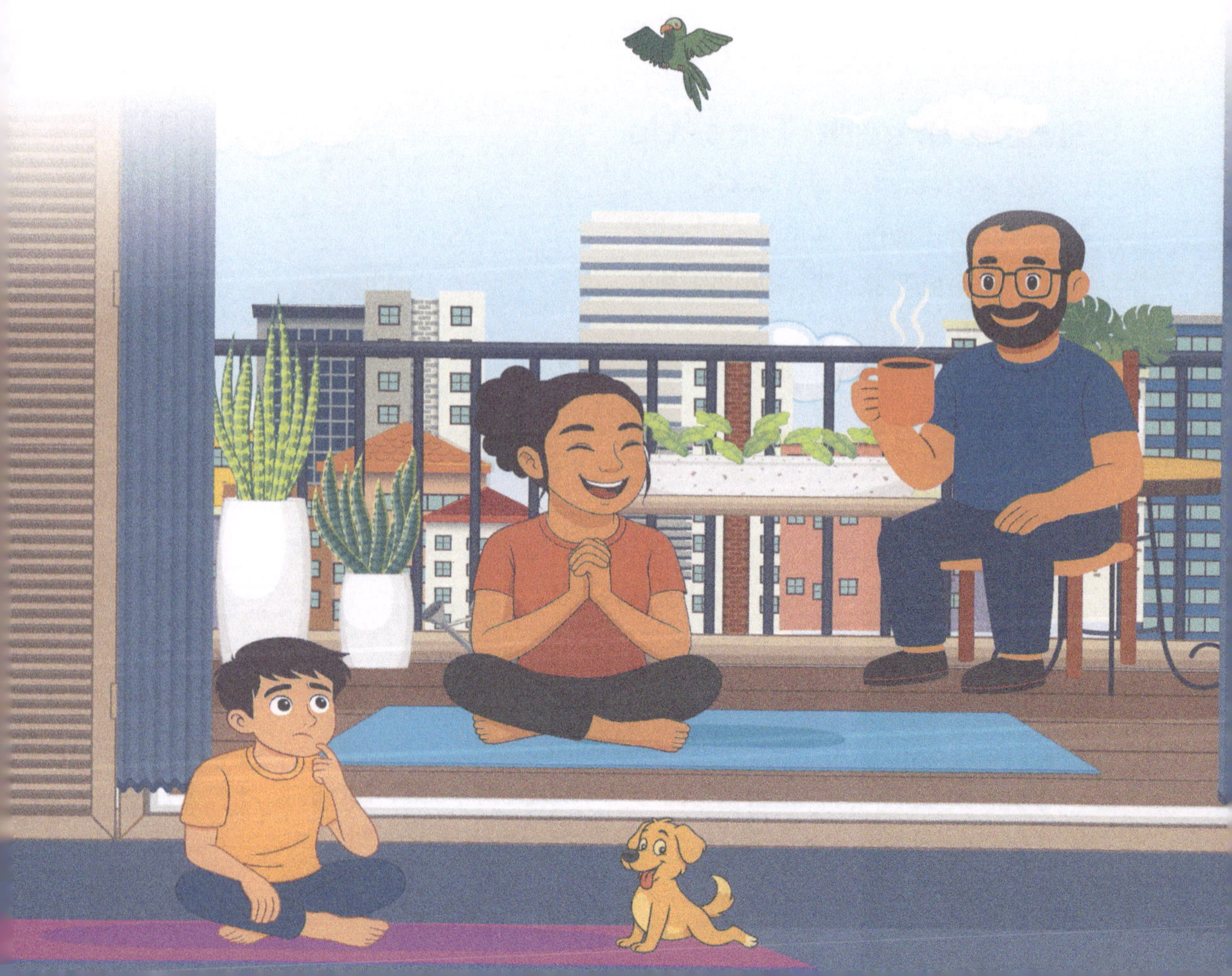

Yoga's Ancient Roots

Uncle Vivek unrolled a scroll. "Yoga began thousands of years ago in India. Early teachers, called rishis, lived in forests and mountains. They studied nature—cats stretching, monkeys climbing, frogs jumping, deer running, kingfisher diving, trees bending in storms, flowers blooming, rivers flowing around rocks. From this, they created postures and breathing techniques."

From Songs to Books

"At first, teachings were passed through songs and stories. Later, they were written in books like the Vedas, Upanishads, and the Bhagavad Gita."

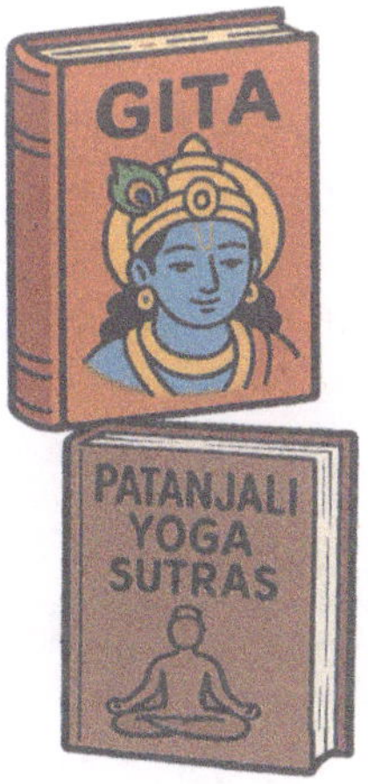

"About 2,000 years ago, a sage named Patanjali organized Yoga into the Yoga Sutras—196 short verses on calming the mind."

He recited: Yogaś citta vrtti nirodhah — (योगश्चित्तवृत्तिनिरोधः) Yoga is the stilling of the mind's fluctuations. "Yoga is the stilling of the mind's ripples."

The Story of the First Yogi

"One legend says Shiva was the first yogi, the Adiyogi. He meditated on a mountain, his being so still that most people walked away. But seven wise Rishis stayed.

Finally, Shiva shared the secrets of Yoga with them. They became the first teachers of the world." There are many other stories, including one that links it to Krishna also.

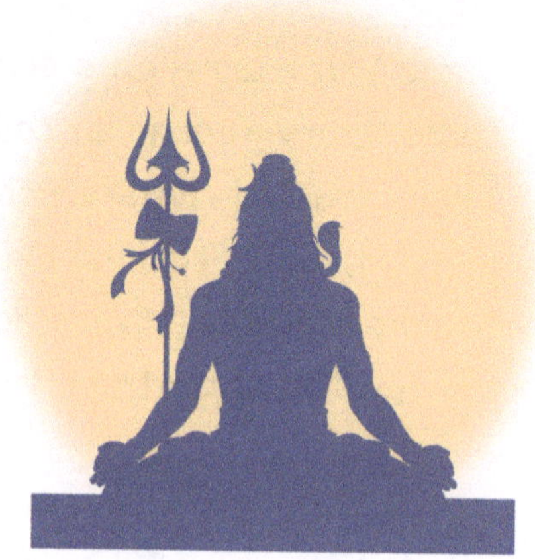

Ravi's eyes widened. "So, Yoga started as a mountain lesson?"

"Yes," Uncle Vivek said. "The story reminds us that patience and curiosity bring wisdom."

Yoga Evolves Through Time

Over centuries, Yoga branched into many forms:

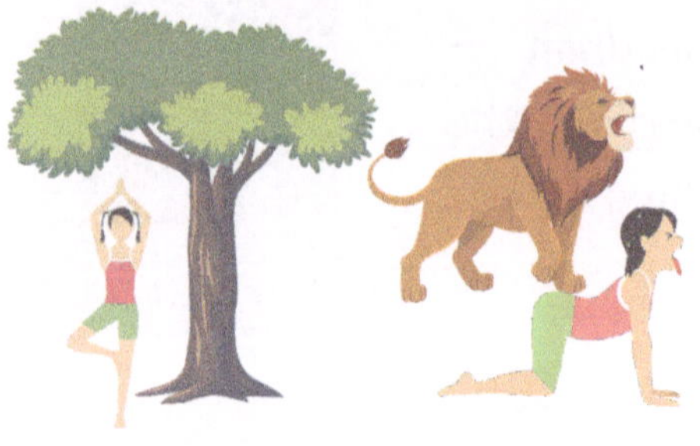

Asanas (poses) inspired by animals and nature.

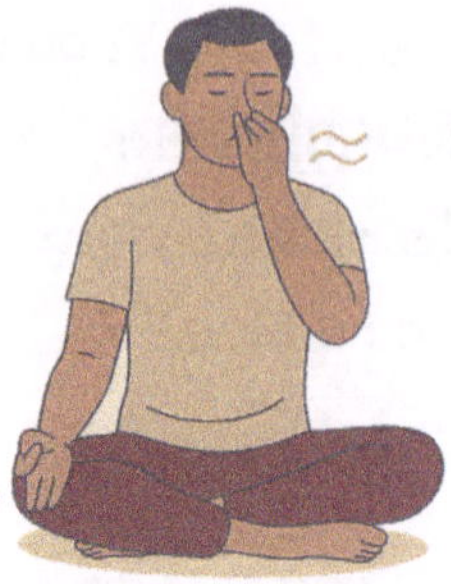

Pranayama (breathing practices).

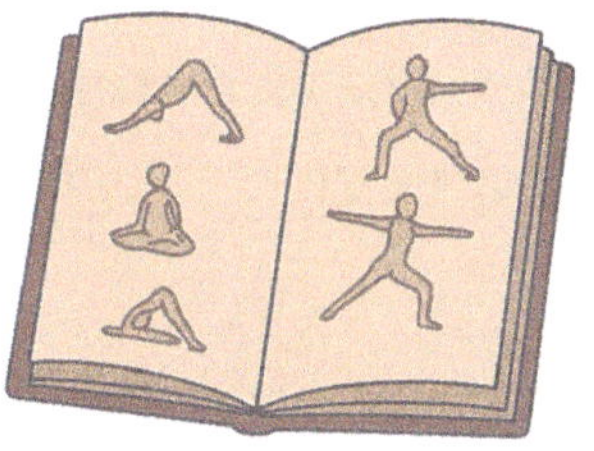

In modern times, teachers like Swami Vivekananda, Maharshi Mahesh Yogi, B.K.S. Iyengar, and Swami Ramdev spread Yoga worldwide.

"Think of Yoga like a tree," Uncle Vivek explained. "All branches come from the same root: balance of body, breath, and mind."

Hatha Yoga texts with dozens of postures.

Symbols and Meanings in Poses

"Why are poses named after animals?" Tara asked. "Because nature was the first teacher."

Tree Pose— rooted yet flexible.

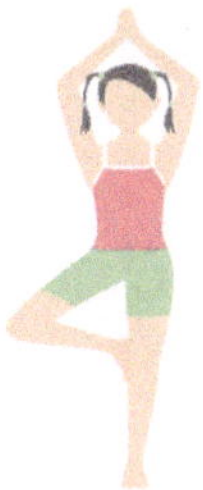

Cobra Pose— strength and openness.

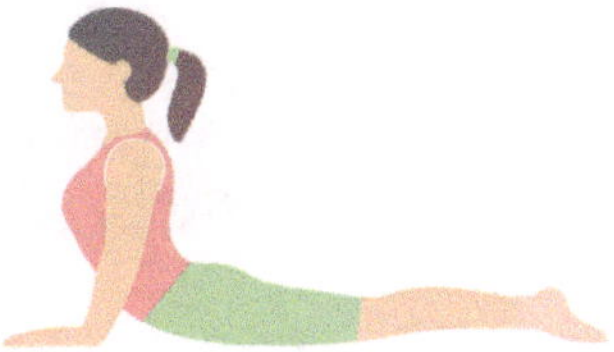

Lion's Breath— courage, letting out fear.

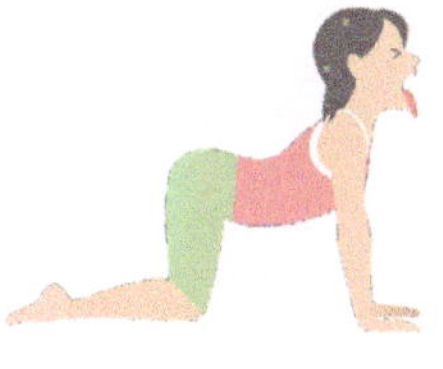

"Animals were the first yogis!" Ravi joked.

"You're right, Ravi!" Uncle Vivek laughed.

Stories as Inner Maps

"Think of Yoga myths like Moana listening to the ocean, or Po finding inner peace," Uncle Vivek said. "They're adventures with hidden wisdom—courage, balance, focus, kindness— superpowers you already have."

COURAGE

BALANCE

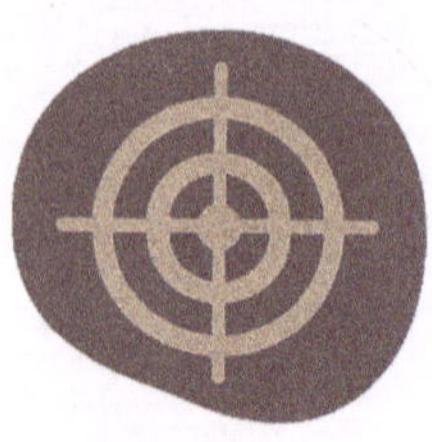

FOCUS

KINDNESS

Try This!

Time-Travel Stretch

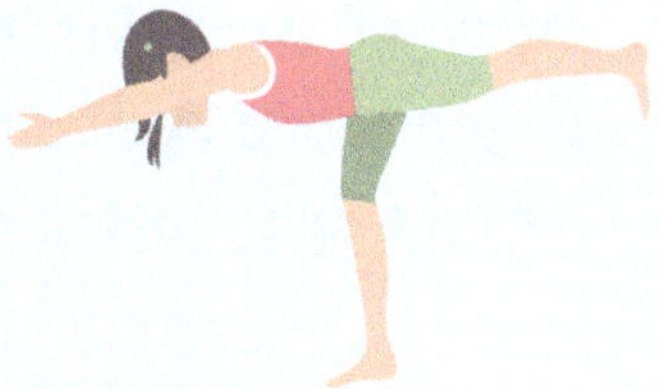

1. Stand tall, arms overhead.
2. Fold forward to the earth.
3. Repeat 3 times, imagining ancient sages by the river.

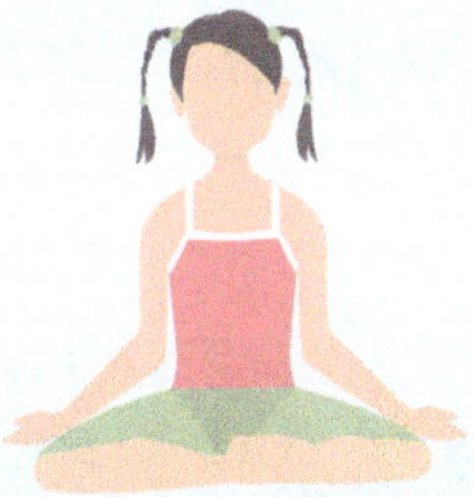

Mind-Wave Pause

1. Sit, close eyes.
2. Inhale calm, exhale distractions.
3. Picture ripples settling on water.

Yoga Safari

1. Cat-Cow (cat stretching).
2. Downward Dog (puppy waking up).
3. Cobra Pose (snake rising).
4. Lion's Breath (roar out worries).

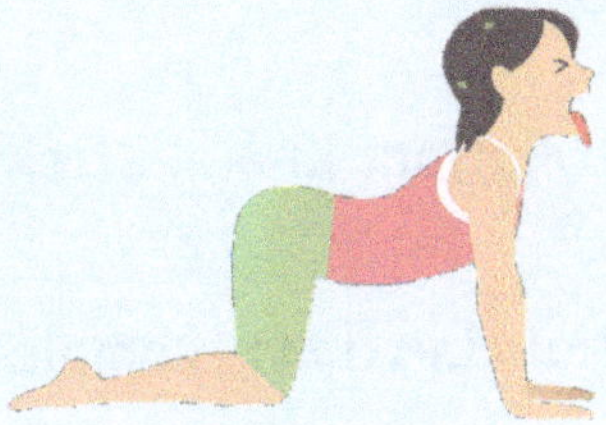

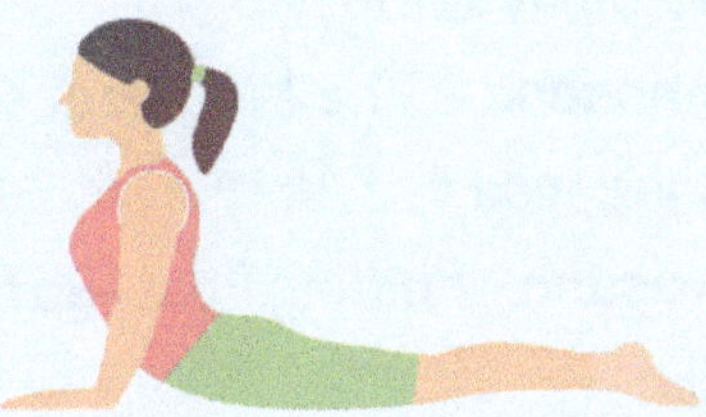

TAKEAWAY

- Yoga began with seekers watching nature.
- Patanjali turned it into clear steps.
- Legends and symbols remind us of inner strength.
- Nature and stories = playful teachers of Yoga.

ADVENTURE QUEST YOGA!

Make up a fun backstory for each pose, use blue scarves for water or wear a cape like a warrior, and take pictures of your coolest poses!

- **Tadasana**- A Warrior standing tall, ready for the quest. Action: Stand firm, reach tall.
- **Vrikshasana**- A steady Tree balancing in the jungle. Action: Balance one foot on the inner thigh/calf.
- **Virabhadrasana I**- The strong Warrior surveys the challenge ahead. Action: Step back, bend front knee, arms up.
- **Nauakasana**- A mighty Boat sailing the ocean waves. Action: Sit, lift feet and chest to form a "V."
- **Bhujangasana**- A graceful cobra raising its hood. Action: Lie on belly, press hands, lift chest.
- **Dhanurasana**- A Warrior aiming for a target. Action: Lie on belly, grab ankles, lift.
- **Simhasana**- The Lion roars in the jungle. Action: Kneel, stick out tongue, roar!
- **Savasana**- Finding Post-Battle Peace. Action: Lie down, completely still.

Part II
Body & Movement

"To infinity... and beyond!"
- Buzz Lightyear, Toy Story

Discover how your body works and grows strong with Yoga.Your body is an amazing machine made of bones, muscles, organs, and trillions of tiny microbial helpers. Yoga keeps this machine strong, flexible, and balanced.

In this part, Ravi and Tara learn:

- How the body is built
- Different styles and paths of Yoga
- The flowing sequence of Sun Salutations
- Super poses that build strength, balance, and flexibility

5. Meet Your Amazing Body

"You're braver than you believe, stronger than you seem, and smarter than you think."
- Winnie the Pooh

Ravi had just rolled out his mat, ready to start, when a sudden thought popped into his head. "Uncle Vivek, how many bones do I even have? It feels like a million when I move!"

Tara bent sideways. "And what about muscles? Which ones help us in Yoga?"

Uncle Vivek chuckled. "Great questions. You're born with about 300 bones, but some fuse together as you grow. By the time you're an adult, you'll have 206 bones making your skeleton."

He pointed to a model of a hand. "Bones protect your brain, heart, and lungs. Your spine and pelvis support every move you make."

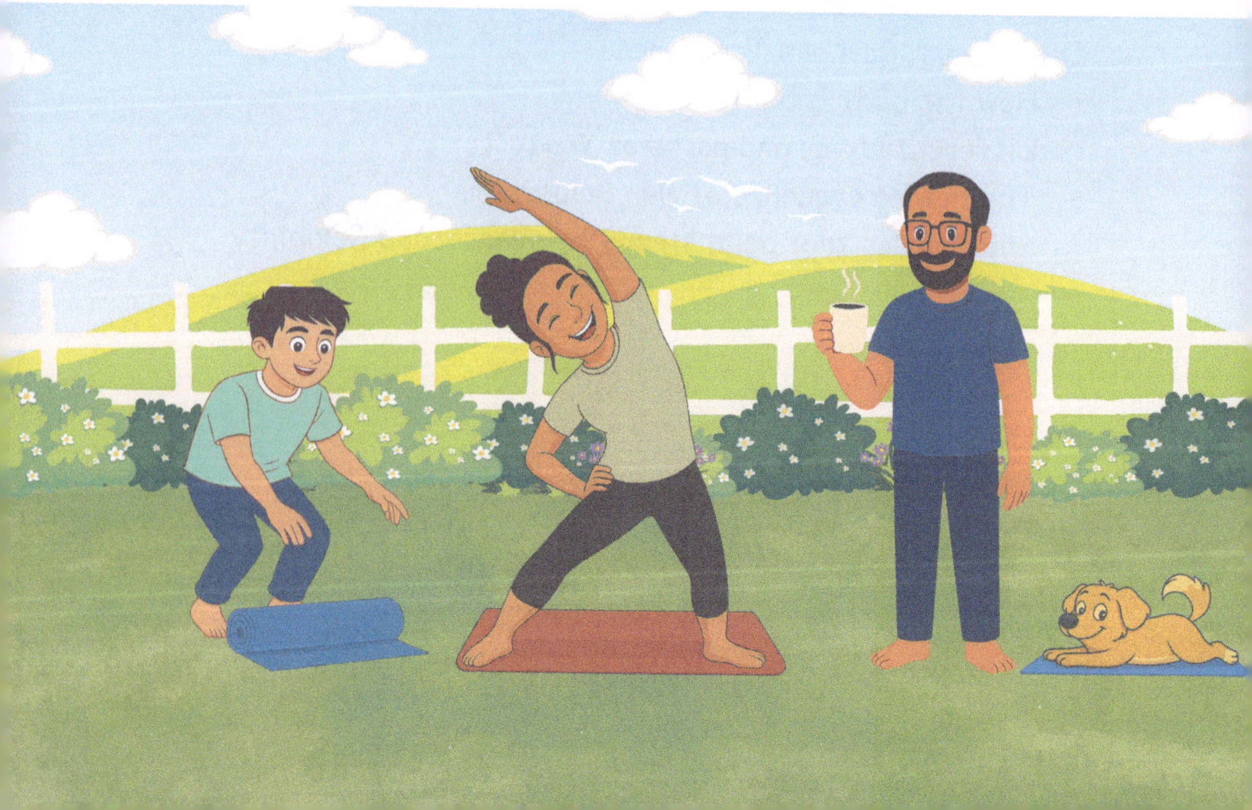

Bones and Muscles: The Super Team

"You also have more than 600 muscles," Uncle Vivek added. "They work in teams— pushing, pulling, and stabilizing your body."

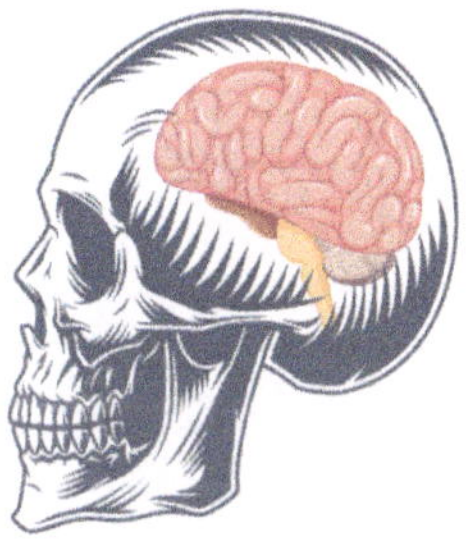

• Skull shields the brain.

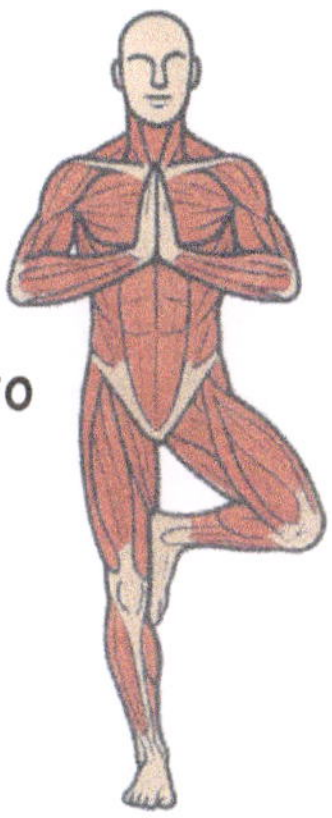

• Muscles move you into Tree Pose or Warrior.

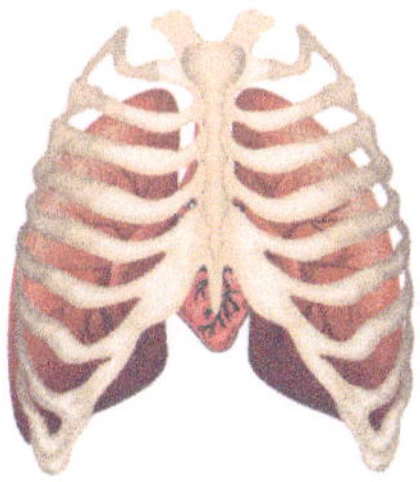

• Ribs guard the heart and lungs.

"Whoa," Ravi said. "So, my skeleton is the armor, and muscles are the movers?"

"Exactly," Uncle Vivek nodded.

Beyond Bones and Muscles

"Your body isn't just a skeleton with muscles," Uncle Vivek explained. "Inside are 11 organ systems."

- Heart pumps blood.
- Lungs bring in oxygen.
- Stomach digests food.

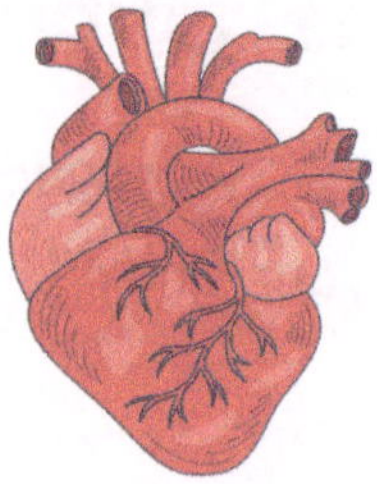

Heart pumps blood

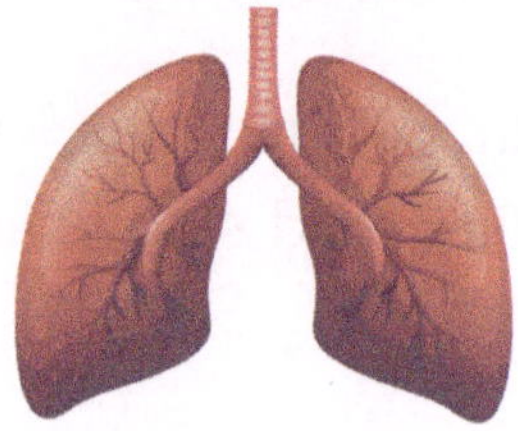

Lungs bring in oxygen

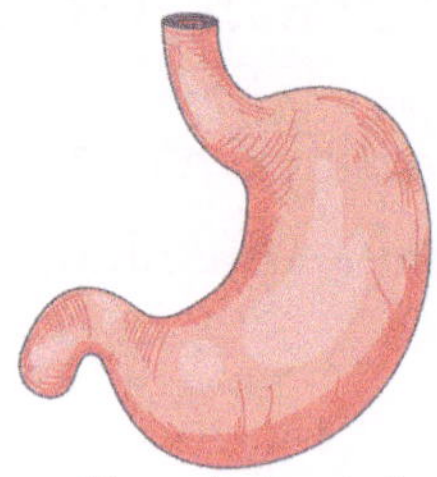

Stomach digests food

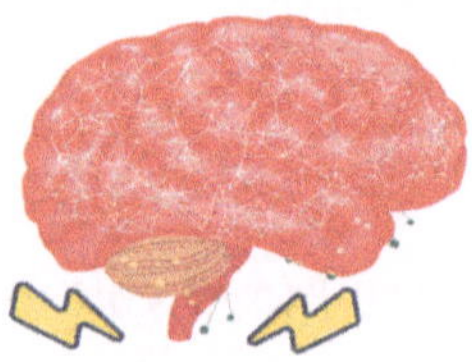

Brain and nerves send signals

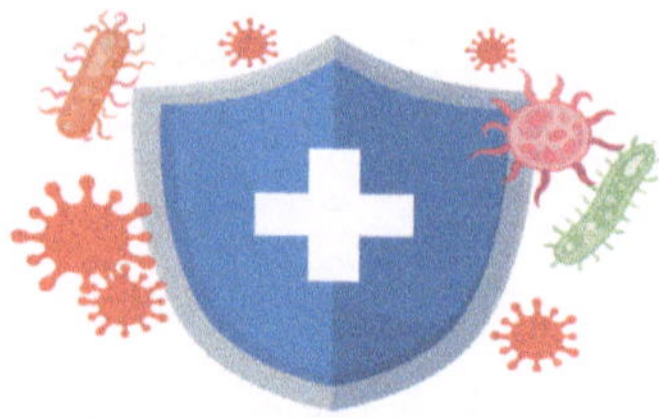

Immune system defends you

- Brain and nerves send signals.
- Immune system defends you.

"They're like teams in a championship league—different jobs, but all play together."

Cellular Cities & Friendly Microbes

"Now zoom in," Uncle Vivek continued. "Your body has about 30 trillion human cells. Each cell is like a tiny city with power plants, factories, and recycling."

"And here's a surprise," he added. "You also carry about 38 trillion microbes—tiny helpers living on your skin and in your gut. They digest food, make vitamins, and protect you from germs."

Ravi gasped. "So, I'm part human, part bacteria?" "Exactly," Uncle Vivek smiled. "You're never alone!"

The Body-Mind Connection

"Yoga shows that body and mind are always talking," Uncle Vivek said.

- **Steady posture** - Calm breath
- **Calm breath** - Clear mind
- **Stressed mind** - tight muscles and shallow breath.

"Yoga helps keep the whole conversation balanced."

FUN FACTS!

- Your body has friendly microbes on your skin and in your gut.
- Gut microbes help you digest food and make vitamins like B and K
- Skin microbes act like natural protectors against harmful germs.
- Everyone has a different microbiome, like a special signature!

Try This!

Bone Touch Game

1. Touch your skull, ribs, hips, knees, and ankles.
2. Say their names out loud.

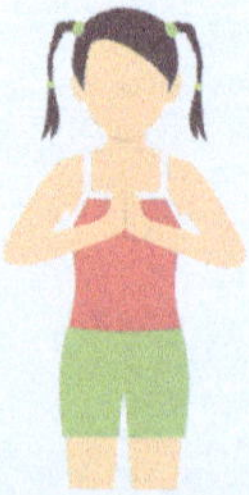

Muscle Power

1. Flex your arms like a superhero.
2. Press palms together at chest.
3. Notice different muscles working.

Breathe & Notice

1. One hand on chest, one on belly.
2. Take 5 slow breaths.
3. Which hand rises first?

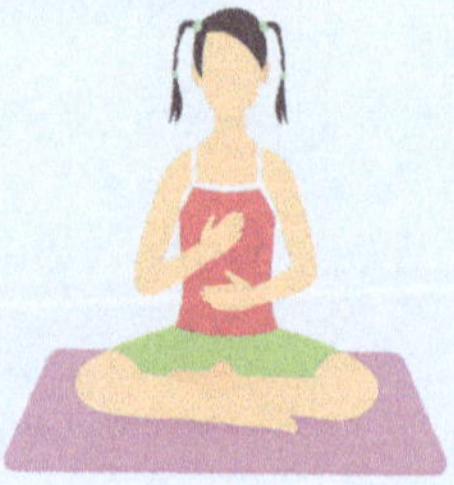

Takeaway

- Bones = framework, muscles = movers, organs = life team.
- Cells and microbes make you a "walking super city."
- Body and mind are always connected.
- Yoga helps keep the whole system balanced.

6. What Type of Yoga Is Best for Kids?

"Talent without working hard is nothing."
- Cristiano Ronaldo

One afternoon, Ravi flopped onto his mat. "I've seen so many kinds of Yoga online. Which one should I try first?"

"Yeah," Tara agreed. "Some look fast, some slow. How do we know what's right for us?"

Uncle Vivek chuckled. "Good question. Yoga has grown into many styles. Let's explore a few and see which feel good for kids like you."

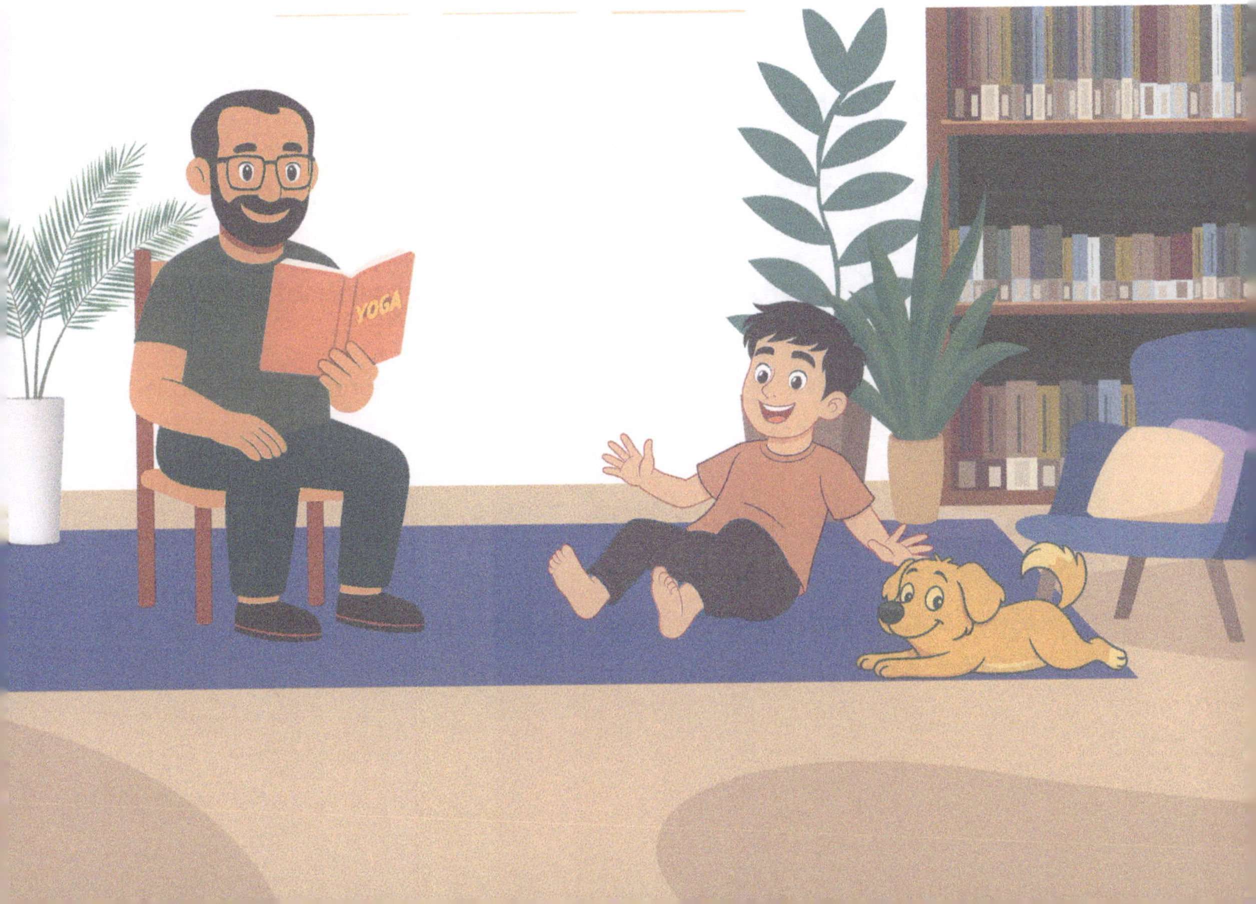

The Eight Steps of Yoga (Ashtanga Yoga)

"Long ago, Sage Patanjali described Yoga in eight steps, like branches of a tree."

- **Yama** - values like kindness and honesty
- **Niyama** - personal habits like cleanliness and gratitude
- **Āsana** - postures for strength and balance
- **Prāṇāyāma** - breathing practices
- **Pratyāhāra** - turning attention inward
- **Dhāraā** - focusing the mind
- **Dhyāna** - meditation
- **Samādhi** - deep peace

"For kids, the first four are most useful: values, habits, poses, and simple breathing. As you grow older, you can explore the deeper steps."

The Four Paths of Yoga

"Swami Vivekananda also explained four main paths," Uncle Vivek continued.

- **Karma Yoga (Action)** — doing the right things without expecting a reward (like Woody in Toy Story).
- **Bhakti Yoga (Love & Devotion)** — showing love and care, trusting the universe without fear or doubt (like Moana singing to the ocean).
- **Jñāna Yoga (Wisdom & Knowledge)** — learning, asking questions, and solving problems (like Hermione in Harry Potter).
- **Rāja Yoga (Focus & Discipline)** — practicing breath, poses, and meditation with patience and discipline (like Po in Kung Fu Panda).

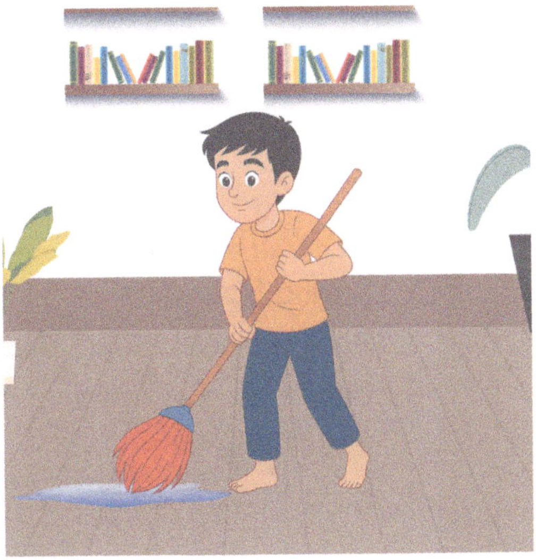

"You come across these paths every day," he added.

Ravi grinned. "So, when I help Mom with chores, that's Karma Yoga?"

"Exactly," said Uncle Vivek.

Modern Styles You Might See

"Today, Yoga is taught in many ways," Uncle Vivek explained.

- **Hatha Yoga** - postures, breathing, meditation
- **Iyengar Yoga** - focus on alignment, uses props
- **Vinyasa Yoga** - flowing poses with breath
- **Kundalini Yoga** - movement, breath, chanting
- **Yin Yoga** - slow, deep stretches

"But beware—some modern fads are just tricks to make money. True Yoga is always about balance of body, breath, and mind."

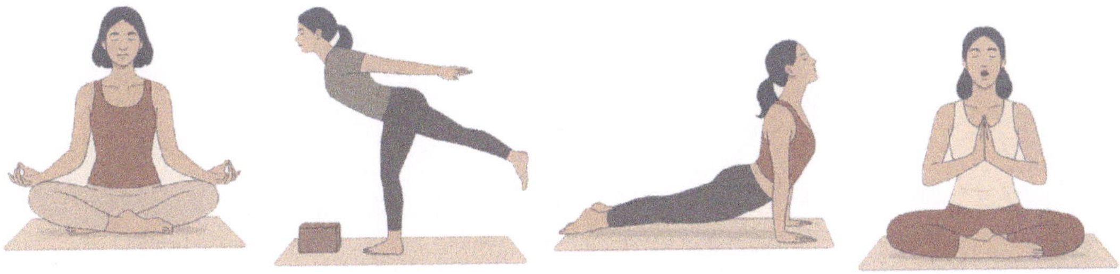

Try This!

Four Mini-Paths

1. Karma Yoga: Do one kind act today.
2. Bhakti Yoga: Sing, draw, or journal with love.
3. Jñana Yoga: Solve a puzzle or build something or learn something new
4. Raja Yoga: Sit still for one minute, noticing your breath.

Takeaway

- Yoga is more than poses—it's a whole lifestyle.
- Patanjali's 8 steps = a guide tree.
- 4 main paths = action, love, wisdom, focus.
- You can create your own "Yoga recipe."

Gratitude Journaling

Think of the moments, people, and qualities that make you feel happy and thankful.

I am grateful for...

7. Sun Salutations - Energy for the Whole Body

"The Sun is the friend of all; it gives light and life to the world."
- Panchatantra

Bathed in gentle morning light, Ravi stretched tall and asked,

"Uncle Vivek, everyone talks about Surya Namaskar. Is it just waving to the Sun?"

Tara laughed. "Like saying 'Good morning, sky!'"

Uncle Vivek smiled. "In a way, yes. Surya means Sun and Namaskar means greeting. Surya Namaskar is a flowing sequence of movements—a thank-you to the Sun for giving us life."

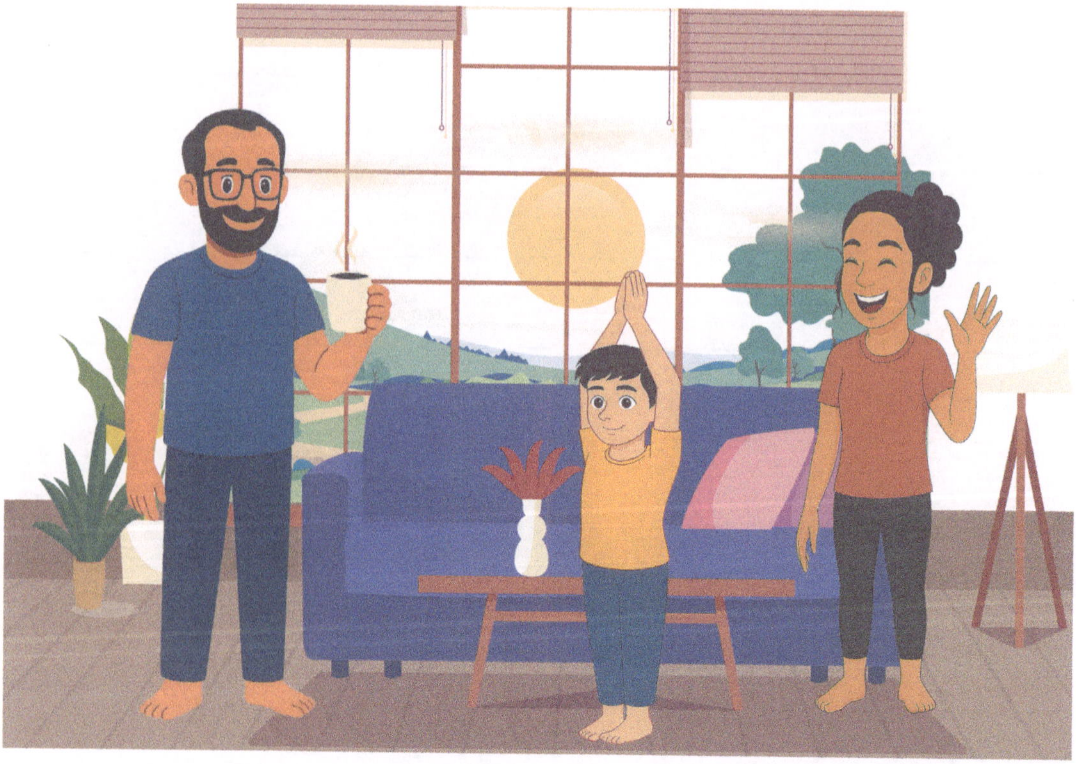

Why the Sun?

"Without the Sun, there'd be no light, food, or warmth," Uncle Vivek explained. "Ancient Yogis honored it as the source of life. Surya Namaskar is both exercise and gratitude."

Tara nodded. "So, it's like charging our body-battery while saying thanks?" "Exactly," Uncle Vivek said.

The 12 Steps of Surya Namaskar

"Each round has 12 steps. It looks long, but once you practice, it flows like a dance."

1. **Prayer Pose** - palms together at heart
2. **Raised Arms Pose** - stretch arms overhead
3. **Forward Bend** - fold down with toes and palms on the ground
4. **Equestrian Pose** - step one leg back
5. **Mountain Pose** - hips high like an upside-down V
6. **Eight-Point Salute** - knees, chest, chin touch the floor
7. **Cobra Pose** - chest up, shoulders back
8. **Mountain Pose again**
9. **Equestrian Pose** - opposite leg forward
10. **Forward Bend**
11. **Raised Arms Pose**
12. **Prayer Pose** - return to stillness

"One cycle = 12 steps. Usually, you repeat it on both sides."

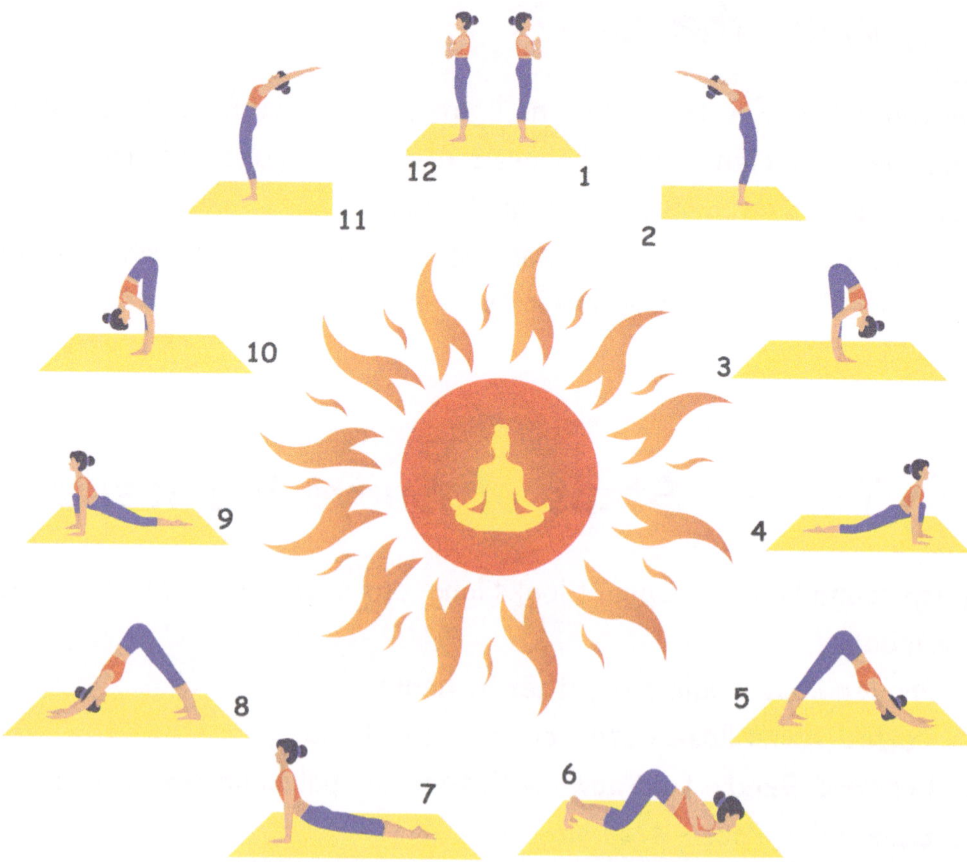

Science of Surya Namaskar

Modern research shows it:

- Strengthens muscles and bones
- Improves flexibility and balance
- Boosts heart and lung health
- Sharpens focus and reduces stress
- Best warm-up exercise.

"Some schools even start the day with Sun Salutations to help kids focus better in class," Uncle Vivek added.

Best Time to Practice

"Surya Namaskar is most powerful at sunrise," Uncle Vivek explained. "But even a few rounds anytime can energize you."
Ravi yawned. "Sunrise? That's too early!"
Vivek laughed. "Then try it later in the morning. The important part is awareness."
Ravi wiped his forehead dramatically. "That was a workout! Do I get Superman powers now?"
"Not Superman powers, but Sun powers!" Uncle Vivek chuckled, "The Sun's strength, calm, and energy to shine."

FUN FACTS!

- Mini cardio: One round gives your heart a gentle morning boost!
- 12-pose power: All major muscles join the "good morning" routine.
- Brain brightener: Forward bends send a quick burst of blood for instant alertness.
- Oxygen recharge: Deep breaths refresh your lungs and energy.

Try This!

Mini Sun Salutation

1. Start with 3 rounds in the morning.
2. Inhale when you stretch up.
3. Exhale when you bend down.
4. At the end, stand still, palms at chest, and whisper "thank you, Sun."

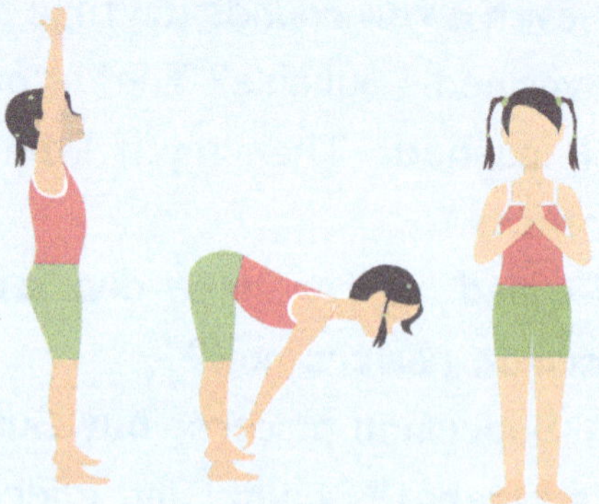

Takeaway

- Surya Namaskar = movement + breath + gratitude.
- It's a natural gym for the whole body.
- Best in the morning or evening, but anytime works.
- Every round = energy boost + thank-you note to life.

8. Yoga for Your Body - Be Strong & Flexible

"The flower that blooms in adversity is the most rare and beautiful of all."
- The Emperor in Mulan

Ravi looked at himself in the mirror and flexed his arms. "I want superhero strength!" he announced.

"And I need flexibility for my dance," Tara added.

Uncle Vivek smiled. "Perfect. Yoga can help you with both. It builds strength and flexibility together. Strong muscles protect your bones, and flexible muscles let you move freely. One without the other isn't enough—balance is the key."

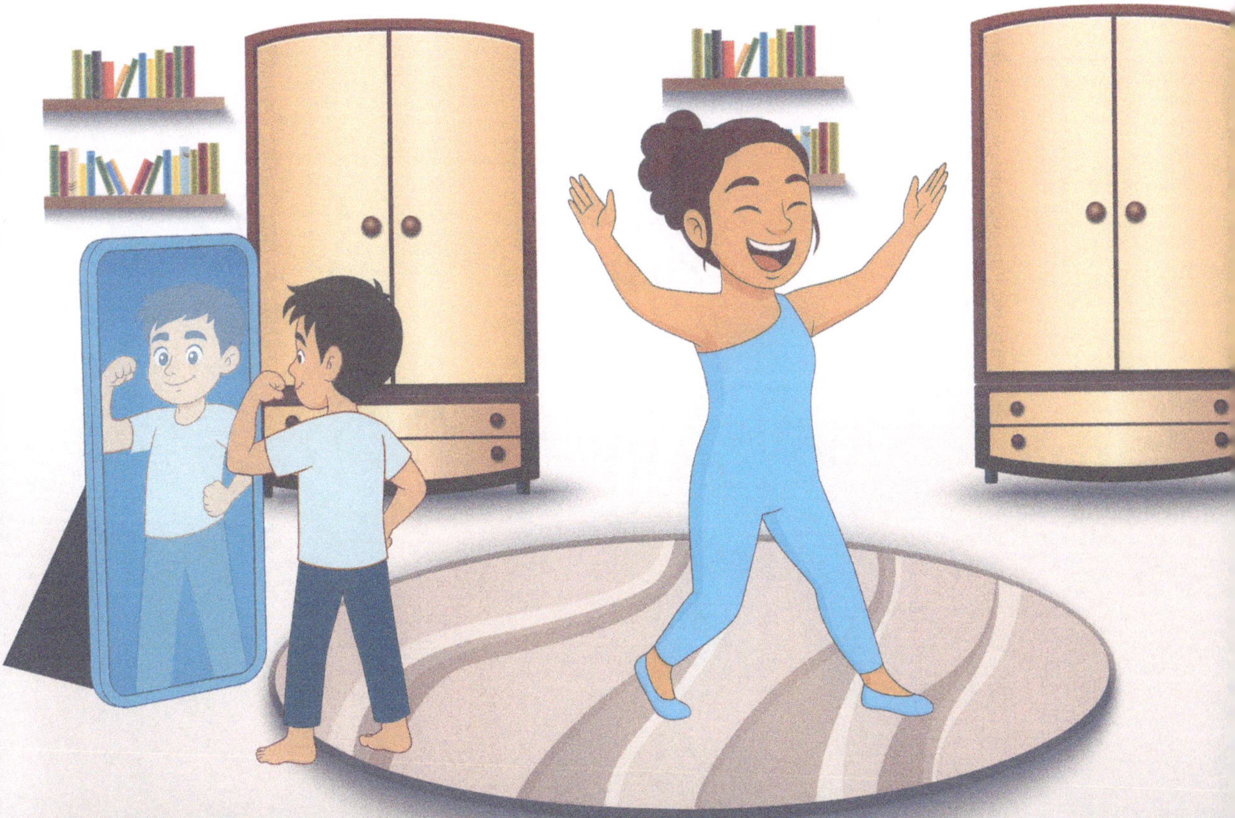

Super Poses for Kids

Uncle Vivek guided them through a few favorites:

1. **Warrior Pose (Virabhadrasana)** - leg and core strength
2. **Tree Pose (Vrikshasana)** - balance and focus
3. **Cobra Pose (Bhujangasana)** - strong back, open chest
4. **Triangle Pose (Trikonasana)** - stretches sides and hamstrings
5. **Bridge Pose (Setu Bandhasana)** - spine and legs strong
6. **Child's Pose (Balasana)** - full-body rest

"These aren't about competition," he reminded them. "They're about feeling steady with every breath."

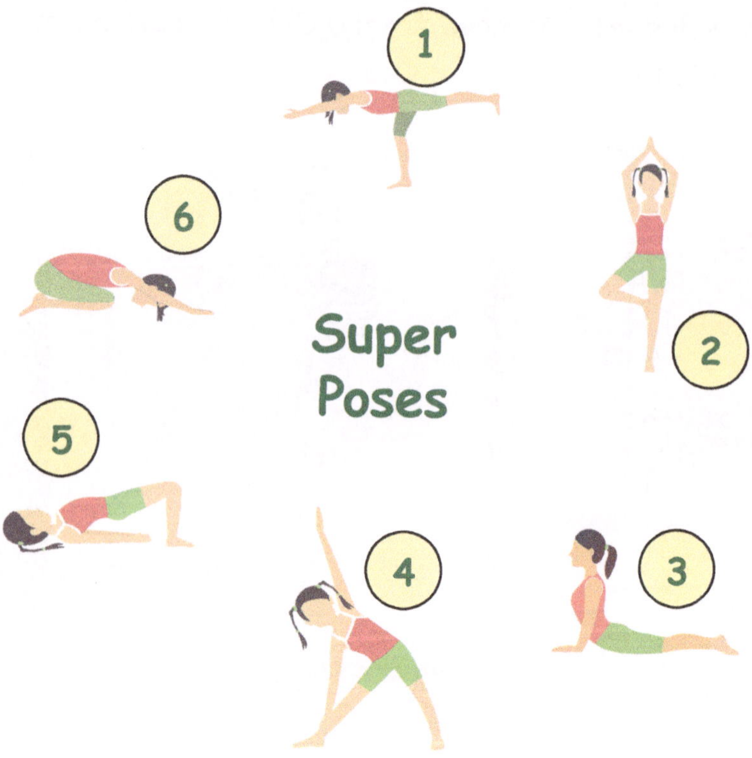

Science Behind the Poses

"When you hold a pose, tiny muscle fibers tear just a little," Uncle Vivek explained. "When they repair, they grow stronger. That's how athletes build muscle—Yoga does it gently."

"And stretching improves blood flow and signals your nervous system to relax. That's why you feel calm after practice."

Ravi grinned in Warrior III. "So, my body upgrades itself?" "Exactly," said Uncle Vivek. "Yoga is self-care disguised as play."

Rest Is Part of Strength - Savasana

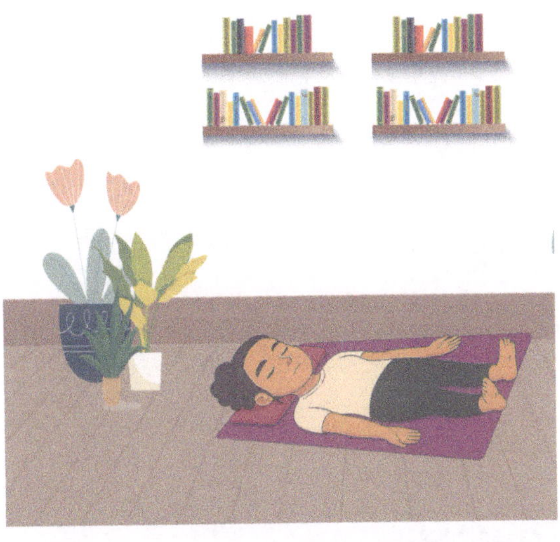

Tara tilted her head. "But what about resting? Is lying down Yoga too?"

"Yes," said Uncle Vivek. "The most important rest is Savasana—lying still at the end of practice. It looks simple, but it lets your body absorb all the benefits."

Ravi flopped onto his mat dramatically. "So first I salute the Sun, then I play dead?"

Tara giggled. "Not play dead—more like recharge mode." My body feels like a team—bones, muscles, breath, and balance all playing together."

Uncle Vivek nodded. "Exactly. Savasana is like plugging in your phone. Stillness gives you quiet strength."

Try This!

Strength Test

1. Come into Bridge Pose.
2. Hold for 5 breaths. Add 2 more next week.

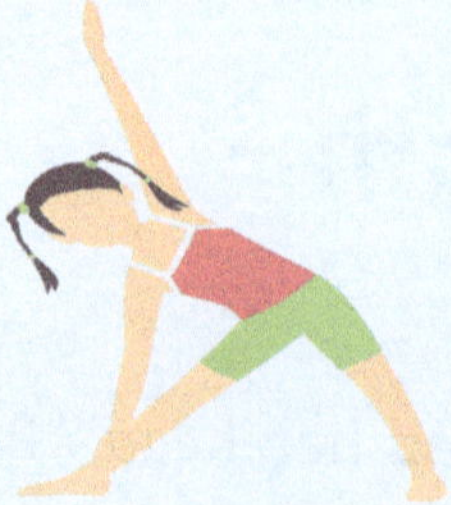

Flexibility Check

1. Stretch into Triangle Pose.
2. Notice how far your hand reaches. Try again tomorrow.

Balance Challenge

1. Stand in Warrior III Pose.
2. Close eyes for 3 seconds.

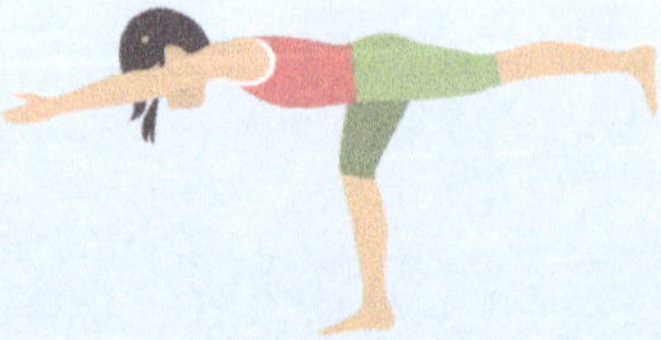

Takeaway

- Strength + flexibility = balance.
- Super poses build both.
- Muscles grow stronger by gentle practice, not force.
- Resting in Savasana is just as important as moving.

Match the pose!

Match the Sanskrit names of the poses with their English ones

1. Trikonasana	A. Tree Pose
2. Virabhadrasana	B. Boat Pose
3. Utkatasana	C. Lion Pose
4. Vrikshasana	D. Downward-Facing Dog Pose
5. Bhujangasana	E. Corpse Pose
6. Nuvakasana	F. Chair Pose
7. Simhasana	G. Cobra Pose
8. Dhanurasana	H. Triangle Pose
9. Adho Mukha Svanasana	I. Bow and Arrow Pose
10. Savasana	J. Warrior Pose

Part III
Breath & Mind

"Remember to breathe. Very important."
– Mr. Miyagi, The Karate Kid

Breath is the secret fuel for focus, calm, and joy
Every inhale is invisible power. Every exhale is a chance to reset.
Yoga teaches how breathing shapes memory, focus, creativity, and happiness.
In this part, you'll discover:

- What prana means and why breath is energy
- The diaphragm and belly breathing
- How Yoga improves memory and creativity
- Why calm breath = a happy heart

9. Breathing in Life - From Prana to Breathwork

"Just keep swimming."
- Dory, Finding Nemo

Ravi took a big sigh after playing his flute.

"Every time I breathe, I feel... alive! But what's really happening inside me?"

Tara added, "Breathing happens automatically. How can this simple thing change everything?"

Uncle Vivek smiled. "In Yoga, we speak of prāna — the life energy flowing through everything. It's somewhat akin to Qi in Chinese traditions. Breath helps this energy move, but prāna is more than just breathing. Each breath brings fresh energy and carries away what we don't need. When we breathe with awareness, we can feel this flow of prāna inside us."

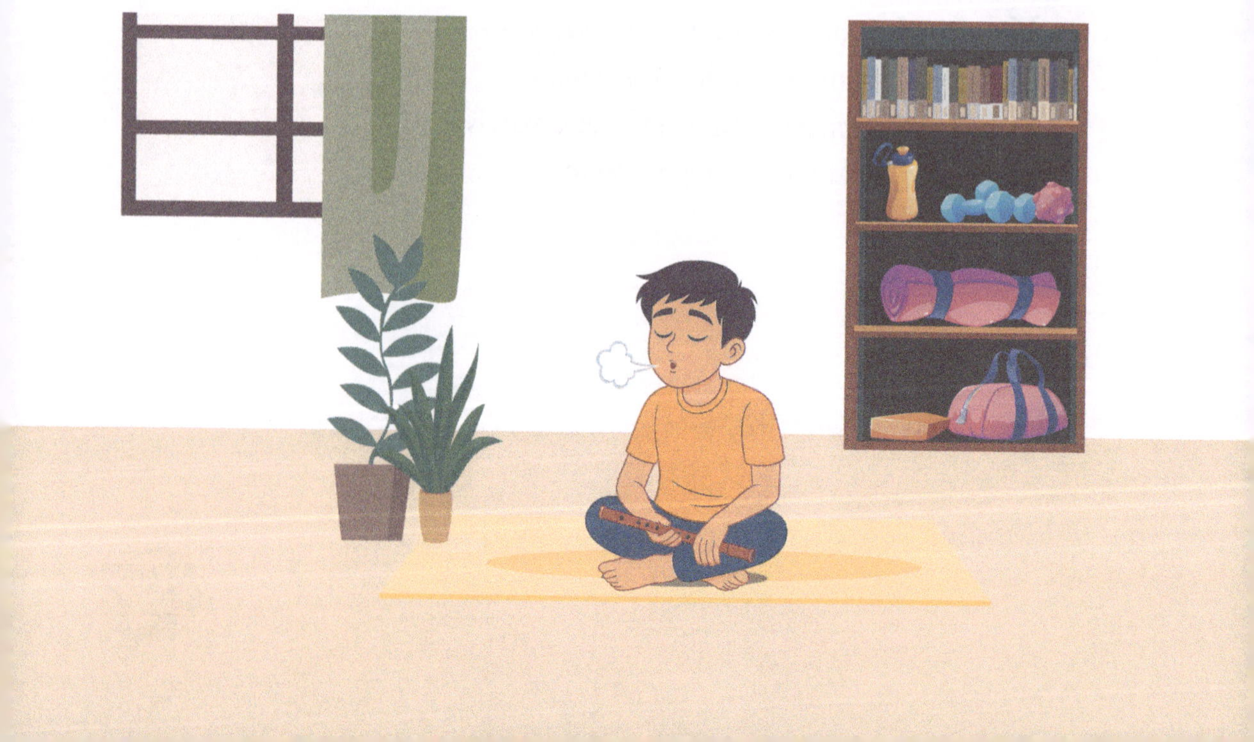

The Science of Breath

"Here's what happens every time you breathe," Uncle Vivek explained, sketching simple diagrams:

1. Inhale - air fills tiny balloons in your lungs (alveoli).
2. Oxygen - jumps into red blood cells.
3. Circulation - blood carries oxygen to muscles, brain, and organs.
4. Energy - oxygen helps cells create ATP, your energy currency.

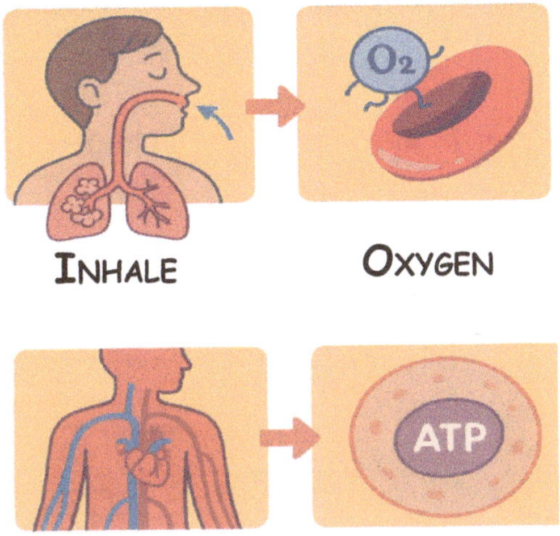

INHALE OXYGEN CIRCULATION ENERGY

"So, every breath is like refueling your body-battery."

Ravi's eyes widened. "Like charging my video game controller?" "Exactly," Uncle Vivek laughed.

Why Breath Matters More Than You Think

"Most people breathe shallow and fast, only using a small capacity of their lungs," Uncle Vivek said. "That makes your heart work harder and your brain foggy."

"But slow, deep breathing calms your nerves, lowers stress hormones, and even improves memory."

Tara nodded. "So, breath is both an invisible fuel and a reset button?"

"Perfectly said," Vivek smiled.

Breath = Superpower

"As you guide your breath with awareness," Uncle Vivek said, "you're not just filling your lungs—you're steering your energy, emotions, and focus."

Ravi leaned back, grinning. "Does it mean that my breath is my hidden superpower?"

"Absolutely," Uncle Vivek nodded. "And now we'll discover the special muscle that makes it all work—the diaphragm."

Try This!

Three-Part Breath (Deep Breathing)

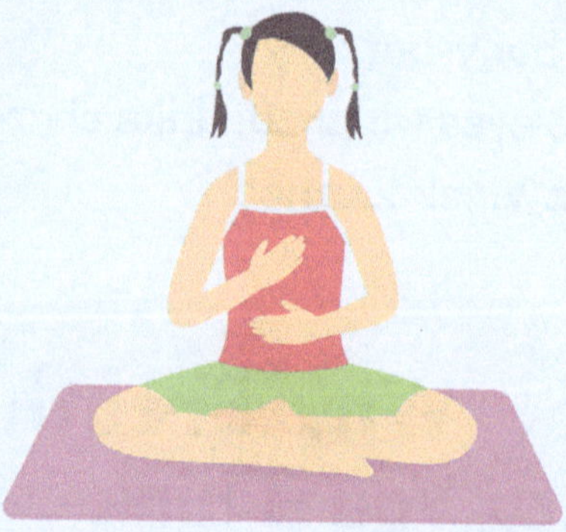

1. Sit tall, hands on chest and belly.
2. Inhale slowly in three parts: belly – chest – upper chest.
3. Exhale in reverse: upper chest – chest – belly.
4. Repeat 5 times.

Breath Awareness Game

1. Close eyes. Count breaths for 1 minute.
2. Slow down and count again.
3. Notice the difference

Takeaway

- Breath = prana, the life force.
- Every inhale charges your body-battery.
- Deep breaths calm stress, sharpen focus, and fuel energy.
- Awareness turns ordinary breath into superpower breath.

FUN FACTS!

- Humans take around 17,000 to 22,000 breaths per day, approximately.
- Inside your lungs are numerous tiny air sacs called alveoli.
- Fish pull in dissolved oxygen from water using their gills.
- A sneeze can blast out air at over 100 km/hr.
- You primarily breathe through one nostril at a time, with dominance switching every few hours.

10. How to Breathe - Diaphragm in Action

"Breathe, you must. Calm, you will be."
- Yoda (Star Wars)

Ravi and Tara sat on their mats, hands on their bellies.

"Uncle Vivek," Tara began, "we practice poses and breaths, but do we really know how to breathe?"

Ravi laughed. "I just do it automatically, like blinking."

Uncle Vivek nodded. "Breathing is automatic. But there's a special way of breathing that makes your body calmer, your heart healthier, and your mind clearer. It's called diaphragmatic breathing (DB), or belly breathing. Babies do it best!"

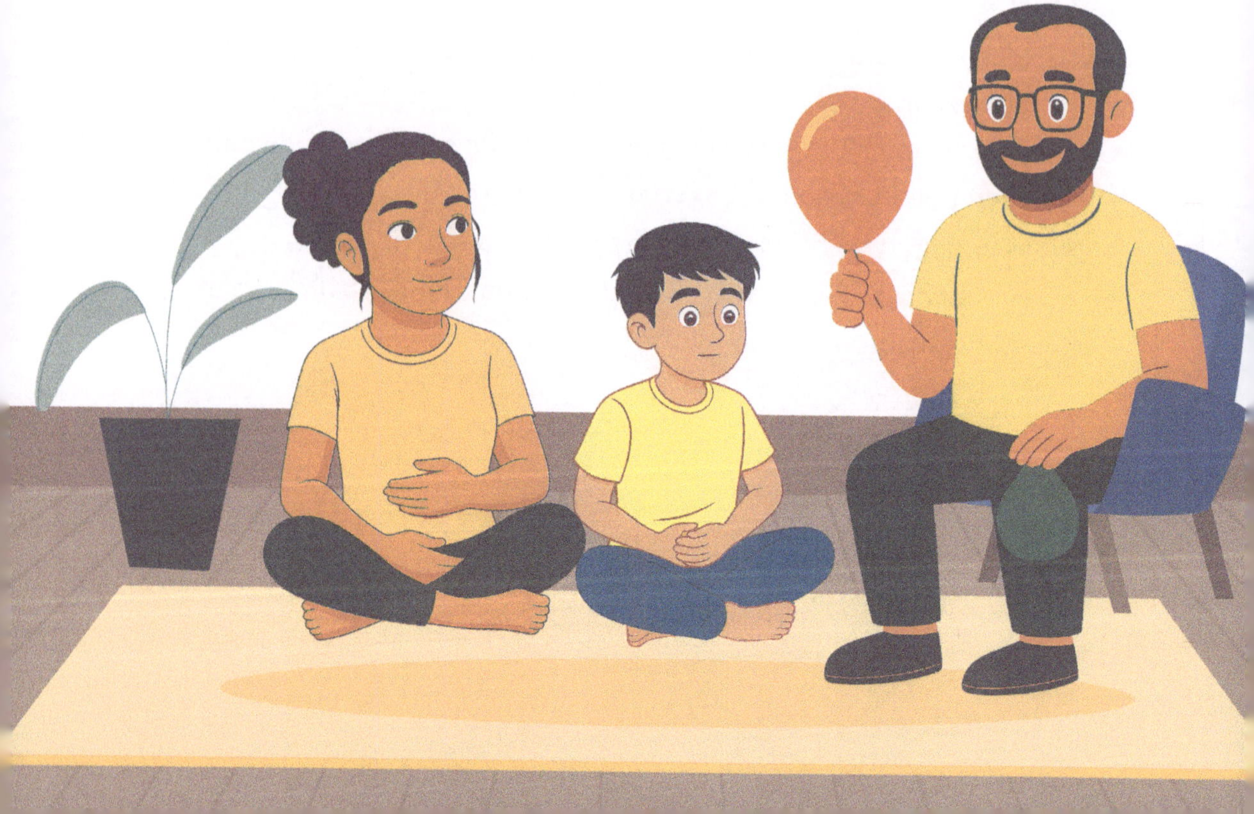

The Baby Secret

"Have you noticed how a baby's tummy rises and falls when they sleep? That's belly breathing. Your belly is like a balloon—it fills when you inhale and softens when you exhale."

"So, my tummy should pop out when I breathe in?" Tara asked.

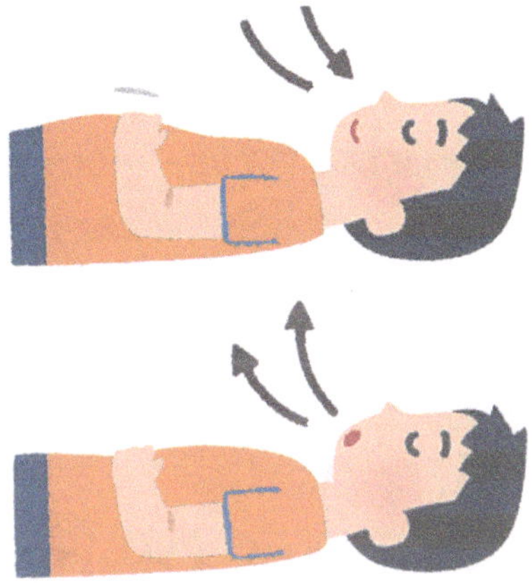

"Exactly," Uncle Vivek said. "That's how nature designed us. Its because the diaphragm pushes the abdominal organs down and out. Many people misunderstand that air goes into the abdomen, hence the clarification.

Why We Forget

"As we grow up, stress, too much sitting, and screen time make us switch to shallow chest breathing. Shoulders go up and down instead of the belly. That tells the body we're stressed—even when we're not

Ravi raised his shoulders dramatically. "Like me while gaming!"

"Right," said Uncle Vivek. "But chest-only breathing makes you tired and jumpy."

The Wave of Breath

"In Yoga, healthy breathing is smooth, deep, and steady, like a gentle wave," Uncle Vivek explained. "When you breathe this way, your heart rhythm steadies, your blood pressure balances, and your mind clears."

Science Connection

Top hospitals like Cleveland Clinic in the USA recommend DB to stay healthy and relaxed.

- Healthy heart - steadier heartbeat
- Strong core - diaphragm supports spine and tummy muscles
- Calm brain - stress hormones go down
- Sharper focus - more oxygen to the brain

"Breathing right makes me stronger, calmer, and smarter?" Ravi grinned. "You're right," Uncle Vivek said.

From DB to Yogic Breathing

"Here's something even cooler," Uncle Vivek continued. "Belly breathing is level one. Full Yogic breathing has three parts:

1. Belly rises (DB).
2. Ribs expand sideways.
3. Chest and collarbone lift.

Exhaling goes in reverse. It's like filling and emptying a glass from bottom to top."

"Whoa," Ravi said. "Is Yogic breathing being turbo mode?" " You can put it that way," grinned Uncle Vivek.

Try This!

The Belly Balloon

1. Sit tall or lie down.
2. Place one hand on chest, one on belly.
3. Inhale slowly—belly rises like a balloon.
4. Exhale—belly softens back.
5. Repeat 5 slow breaths.

Tara whispered, "It feels like my body is melting into the mat!"

Three-Part Breath

1. Place one hand on belly, one on ribs.
2. Inhale: belly rises — ribs expand — chest lifts.
3. Exhale: chest — ribs — belly.
4. Repeat 5 times, like a smooth wave.

"That feels like the ocean moving through me!" Tara exclaimed.

"That's Yogic breathing," Uncle Vivek smiled. "The bridge between body, breath, and mind."

TAKEAWAY

» Babies breathe best—belly first.
» Shallow chest breathing = stress mode.
» DB = calmer body, clearer mind, stronger heart.
» Yogic breathing = full wave, turbo mode.

11. Yoga for Your Mind: Focus & Memory Boost

"The mind is everything. What you think, you become."
— Buddha

It was a quiet evening. The sky outside glowed orange as Ravi and Tara sat at their study table. Books were spread everywhere, and even their pencils looked tired.

Ravi groaned over his math notebook, feeling overwhelmed.

"I've got a big test tomorrow. Can Yoga really help me concentrate?"

"And can it help me remember what I study?" Tara added.

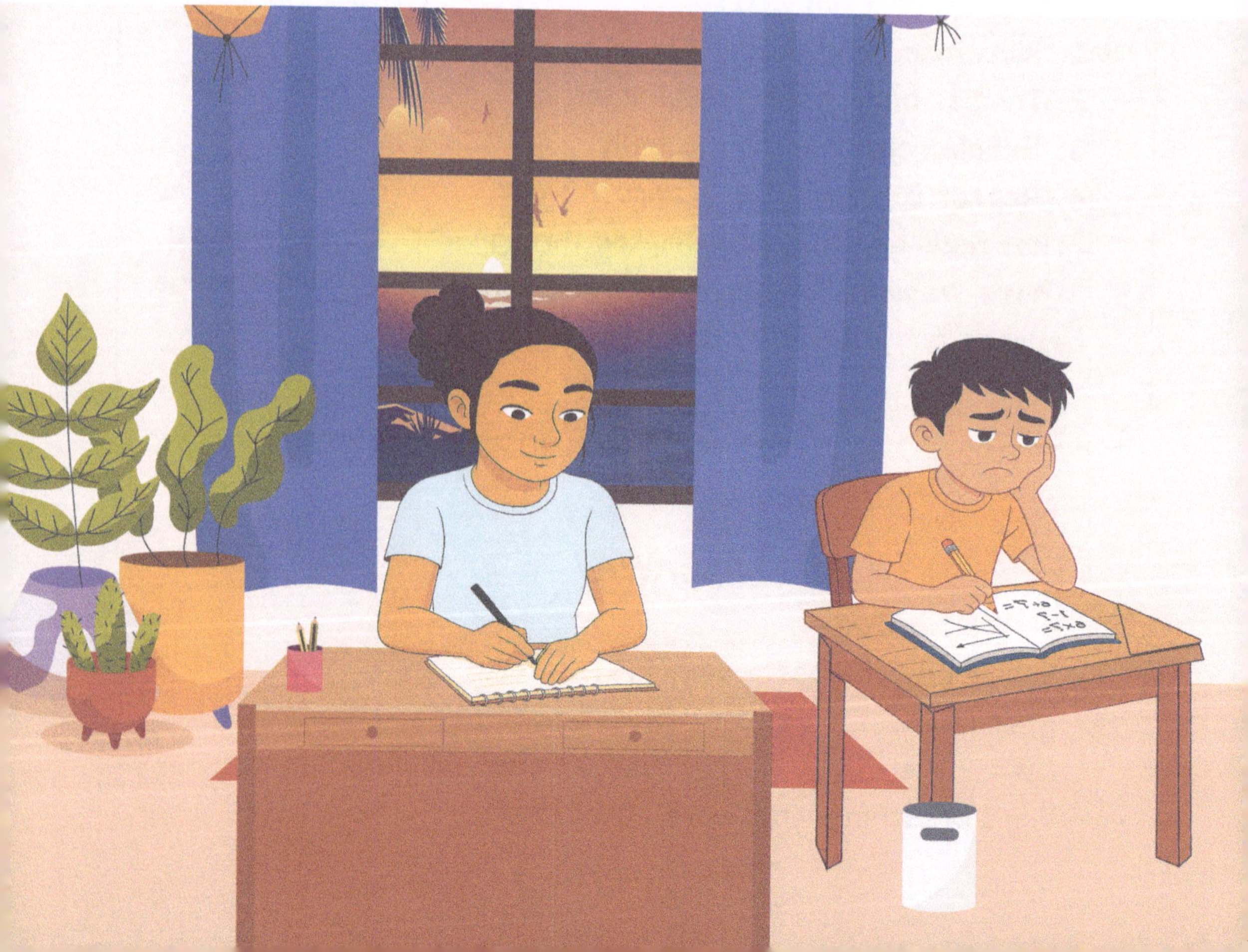

Uncle Vivek smiled. "Yoga won't solve equations for you, Ravi. But it can tune your brain and your mind like updating the software and upgrading the hardware of a computer."

Ravi frowned. "Brain and mind? Aren't they the same?"

Uncle Vivek shook his head. "Not quite. The brain is the organ inside your head. It sends messages, stores information, and controls your movements. The mind is the invisible part that thinks, feels, and remembers. The mind uses the brain, just like a musician plays an instrument."

Tara leaned back in her chair. "Uncle, once I heard someone say Chitta Bhūmi. Is that about the mind too?"

"Yes," he said gently. "It helps us understand how the mind behaves."

He continued, "Sometimes the mind is like a donkey, carrying old worries even when they are not needed.

Sometimes it becomes a monkey, jumping from one thought to another.

Sometimes it is a butterfly, settling for a moment and then drifting away.

And sometimes the mind becomes like a candle flame, steady and clear."

Ravi nodded slowly. "So Yoga helps the mind become like the candle flame?"

"That is the idea," Uncle Vivek said. "When the mind steadies, the brain works better, and studying feels easier."

Tara nodded. "So Yoga helps both, mind and brain?"

Uncle Vivek smiled. "Exactly. A calm mind helps the brain work better. Yoga keeps both clear and connected." Tara thought for a moment.

"We can see inside our body with an X-ray, but how can we see inside our mind?"

Uncle Vivek laughed softly. "Good question, Tara. If X-rays are for the body, Yoga is like a mind-ray that helps us understand ourselves better. When we breathe slowly and watch our thoughts, we begin to 'see' what's happening inside." He continued, Yoga helps us awaken awareness — the gentle light that lets us see what's happening inside. This light of awareness is what we call consciousness.

Ravi grinned. "So Yoga helps us look inside our mind?"

Uncle Vivek nodded. "Yes — that's where meditation comes in."

Meditation = Playground for the Mind

"Yoga isn't only movement," Uncle Vivek continued.

"It also means sitting quietly, breathing slowly, and watching thoughts float by like clouds."

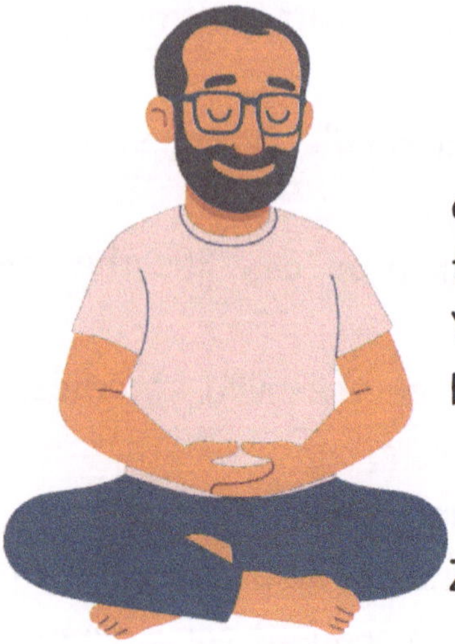

Tara smiled. "Meditation is just like a calm playground for the mind !"

"Correct," said Uncle Vivek. "In Japan and China, they call it Zen. The word comes from dhyāna, which means deep meditation. Yoga and Zen use different names, but both bring peace inside."

Ravi laughed. "Look at me, Tara! When I meditate, I'm doing Yoga — and a little Zen too!"

Focus: Closing Extra Tabs

"Think of your brain like a computer with too many tabs open," Uncle Vivek explained. "Crowded thoughts and worries slow it down. Yoga helps you close extra tabs and focus on one thing at a time."

Ravi nodded eagerly. "Like stopping lag in a video game?" "Exactly," said Uncle Vivek.

Memory: Upgrading Your RAM

"Controlled breathing and meditation strengthen the hippocampus — that's the brain's memory center," Uncle Vivek explained. "It's like adding more RAM so you can store and recall better."

Ravi asked, "So Yoga is like a memory upgrade?"

"Perfect comparison," Uncle Vivek said with a smile.

Creativity: A Clean Desktop

"A calm mind is like a clean desktop," said Uncle Vivek. "When it's uncluttered, new ideas appear."

Tara clapped her hands. "That's why I get story ideas after meditation!" "Indeed, Tara," he nodded. "Creativity grows best in quiet spaces."

Brain vs. Mind —

Brain:

- The brain is part of your body.
- It's made of billions of nerve cells called neurons.
- It controls movement, senses, and memory.

Mind:

- The mind is not physical — it's where thoughts, emotions, and imagination live.
- It uses the brain to think, feel, and remember.
- You can't see it, but you can sense it through awareness.

Yoga connects the two.
When the breath is calm, the brain relaxes.
When the mind is peaceful, the brain performs at its best.

Try This!

Equal Breathing for Focus

1. Sit tall.
2. Inhale for 4 counts, exhale for 4 counts.
3. Repeat 10 breaths before studying.

Memory Test

4. Read a short list of words.
5. Do one minute of belly breathing.
6. Try to recall the words — notice the difference!

Creative Spark

7. Sit quietly for three minutes.
8. Write or draw the first idea that comes to mind.

Takeaway

- Yoga helps focus by closing "extra tabs."
- Breath and meditation boost memory like a RAM upgrade.
- Calm minds are creative minds.

12. Yoga for Your Heart & Happiness

"Laughter is ten times more powerful than screams."
– Sulley, Monsters, Inc.

Ravi took a deep breath, resting his hand over his heart.

"I've heard people say Yoga is good for the heart. But how can stretching and breathing make it healthier?"

"And does it really make us happier too?" Tara asked.

Uncle Vivek smiled. "Yes, and yes. Let's see how Yoga cares for both your physical heart and your emotional heart."

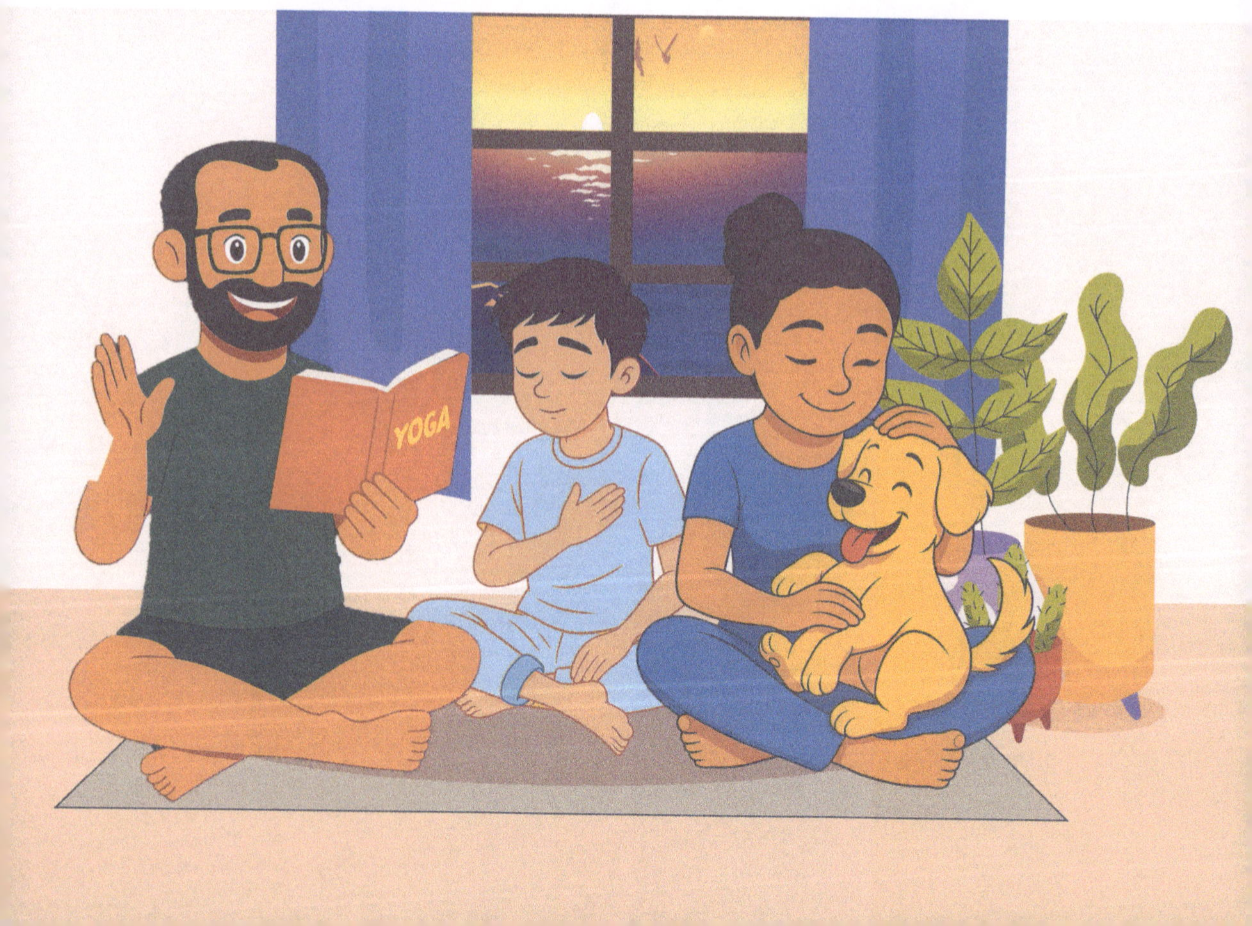

Heart Health: A Steady Engine

"Think of your heart as an engine that never rests. It beats about 100,000 times a day!" Uncle Vivek explained.

"When you practice Yoga, your heart rate becomes smoother. Scientists call it heart rate variability (HRV)—the tiny differences between beats. A flexible HRV = a healthier, calmer heart."

"Does Yoga make my heart more flexible, like my muscles?" Ravi asked.

"That's right, strong boy!" Uncle Vivek cheered.

Happiness Hormones

"Yoga also changes brain chemistry," Uncle Vivek added. "It boosts natural feel-good chemicals: endorphins, serotonin, and dopamine. These lower stress and lift mood."

Tara nodded. "That explains the happy rush after Yoga class."

"Yes," he said. "Yoga lowers cortisol (the stress hormone) and raises happiness hormones. Less stress + more joy = balance."

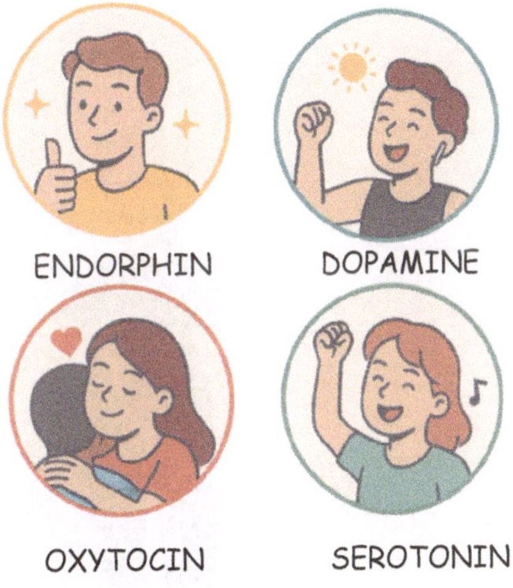

Mind-Heart Connection

Our mind thinks, but our heart feels. Sometimes they agree — and sometimes they argue! Yoga helps them become friends again, so we can feel calm and whole inside.

Uncle Vivek placed his hand on his chest. "Your heart isn't just a pump. It also reacts to emotions. Think about how your chest feels heavy when you're sad, or light when you're happy."

He guided them through a gentle backbend (Camel Pose), then curled into Child's Pose. "Opening your chest improves circulation and makes space for emotional release."

Ravi frowned. "Uncle, what happens when I feel my heart heavy?"

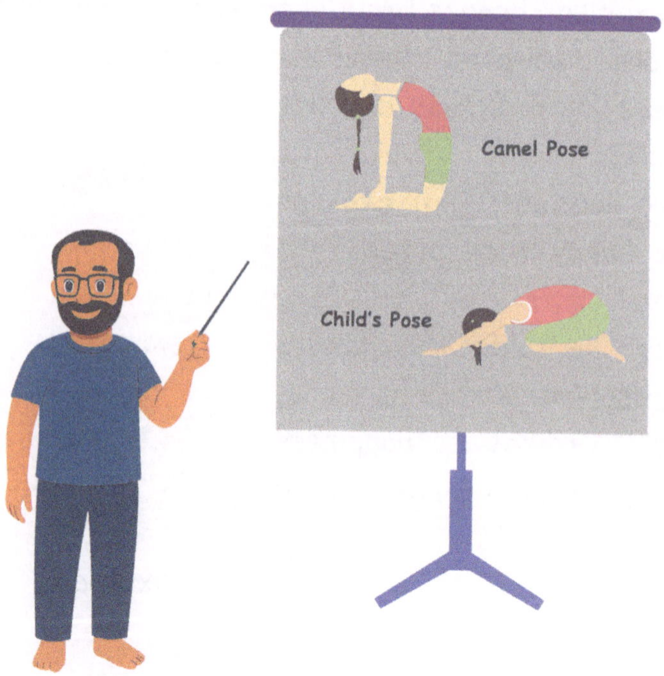

Uncle Vivek nodded gently. "That's your emotions speaking, Ravi. When you feel sad, worried, or scared, your heart muscles tighten a little — that's why it feels heavy or closed."

Tara thought for a moment. "Like in that movie Inside Out, when Sadness made everything feel blue and Joy tried to cheer everyone up?"

Uncle Vivek smiled. "Exactly, Tara! That movie shows how different feelings live inside us — just like little friends in our mind and heart. When one takes over, we feel it in our body too. Sadness can make the heart feel heavy; Joy makes it light and warm."

He placed a hand on his chest again. "Yoga helps all those emotions live together peacefully. When we breathe deeply and open our chest, we give every feeling space to move and settle. That's how the heart and mind become friends again."

Ravi brightened. "So when I feel heavy-hearted, I can take slow breaths to make room for Joy?"

Uncle Vivek chuckled. "Yes, Ravi. That's the Yoga way — letting every emotion have its moment, then returning to balance."

Try This!

Heart Rate Check

1. Count your pulse for 30 seconds.
2. Do 3 Sun Salutations.
3. Count again—notice the change.

Mood Lift Flow

1. Do Bridge Pose for 5 breaths.
2. Rest in Savasana.
3. Notice your mood afterward.

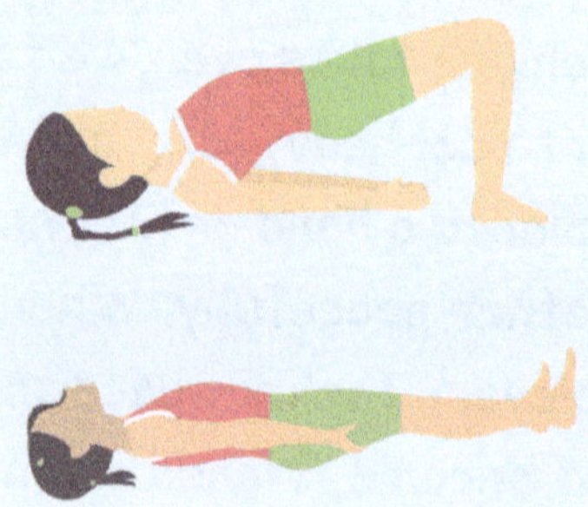

Heart-Opening Cycle

1. Alternate Camel Pose and Child's Pose 5 times.
2. Imagine inhaling sunshine, exhaling worries.

Takeaway

- Your heart is an engine—Yoga keeps it flexible and calm.
- Yoga lowers stress and boosts happiness chemicals.
- Chest-opening poses = sunshine for your heart.

Part IV
Balance & Science

"Body and mind must work together. If one is weak, the other cannot win."
– Novak Djokovic (tennis)

Explore the inner maps of Yoga and how science explains them
Ancient Yogis described five layers of being, five vital winds, spinning energy centers, and the sound of Om. Modern science is now finding proof of many of these insights.

In this part, Ravi and Tara explore:

- The five koshas (layers of being)
- The five pranas (winds within)
- Chakras along the spine
- Yoga as both ancient wisdom and modern science

13. Layers of Being - The Pancha Kosha

"What is essential is invisible to the eye."
- The Little Prince

Tara carefully opened a Matryoshka doll, revealing smaller ones nested inside. Ravi watched, intrigued.

"Uncle," he asked, "we have learned about bones, breath, and even the brain. But is there more to us than body parts?"

"Yes," Uncle Vivek said. "Ancient teachers described a human being as having five layers, called the Pancha Kosha. Think of them like onion layers — or like your Matryoshka dolls. Each doll sits inside another, and each layer brings you closer to your true self."

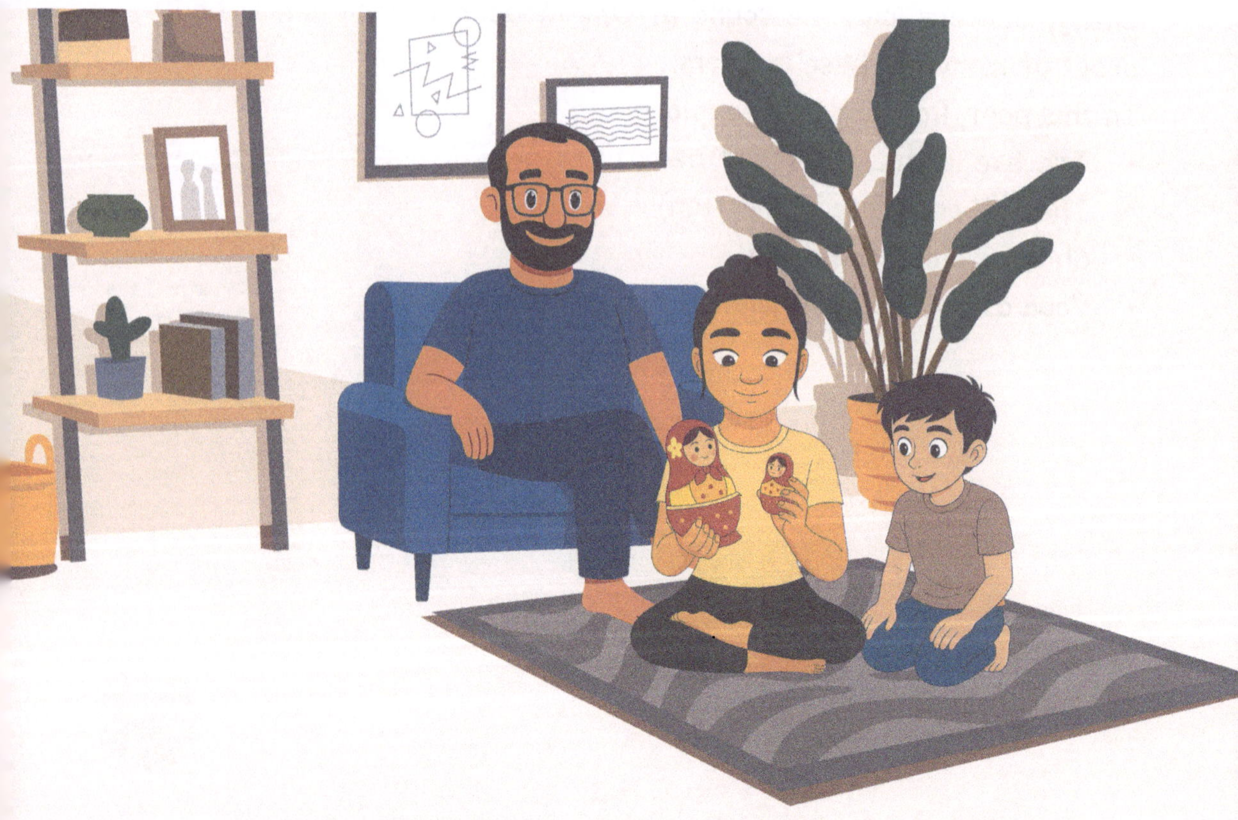

The Five Layers

Uncle Vivek counted on his fingers:

1. **Physical Layer (Annamaya Kosha)** — the outer doll, your body made of food: bones, muscles, skin.
2. **Energy Layer (Pranamaya Kosha)** — the next doll, your breath and vital energy.
3. **Mind Layer (Manomaya Kosha)** — your thoughts, feelings, and everyday reactions.

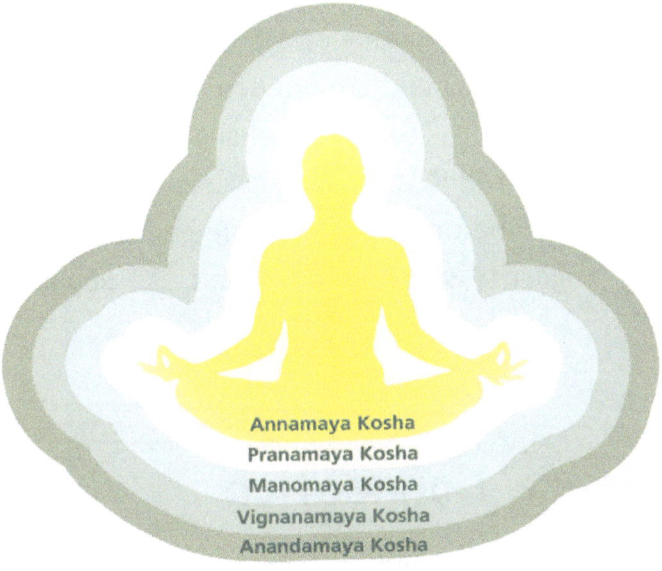

4. **Wisdom Layer (Vijnanamaya Kosha)** — your inner understanding that helps you choose what is right.
5. **Bliss Layer (Anandamaya Kosha)** — the innermost doll, the quiet sense of peace

and joy when you feel safe and connected.

Ravi widened his eyes. "So I'm like... five-in-one?"

"We all are," Uncle Vivek said with a smile. "Yoga helps us understand each layer and care for all of them."

Education Connection

"Schools today know that real education means all-round development," Uncle Vivek said. "It is not only about remembering facts. It is about helping every part of a child grow."

He pointed to the Matryoshka dolls again. "The Pancha Kosha reminds us what a complete education should nurture:

- A strong and healthy body
- Steady breathing and balanced energy
- Stable emotions
- Clear thinking and wise choices
- An inner sense of joy and confidence"

He paused for a moment. "Swami Vivekananda also said that education must bring out the fullness already present in every child. Not just the brain, not just the body — the whole person."

"That is why Yoga fits so well," he added. "It supports growth in all five layers."

Science Connection

"Science uses different words," Uncle Vivek continued. "It talks about body systems, brain networks, cognition, and psychological well-being. Yet the understanding is very close to what the sages taught."

He tapped the smallest doll. "Health and growth are not only about the physical body. They include emotional balance, thoughtful decisions, creativity, and the ability to feel calm and happy."

Tara nodded. "So Yoga helps every layer, not just muscles and bones."

"Well said, Tara," Uncle Vivek replied. "It helps the whole child — inside and out."

Try This!

Layer Awareness

1. Close eyes.
2. Notice your body (physical).
3. Notice your breath (energy).
4. Notice feelings/thoughts (mind).
5. Ask: "What feels right?" (wisdom).
6. Rest in stillness (bliss).

TAKEAWAY

» You have five layers: body, energy, mind, wisdom, joy.
» Education should nurture all five.
» Yoga is the practice that keeps them balanced.

14. Winds Within - Understanding the Five Energies

"The wind is calling... and I must follow."
- Frozen II

One breezy evening, Ravi watched the curtains dance in the wind.

Uncle Vivek smiled. "Remember how we talked about prāna — the life energy that moves through everything? In Yoga, this energy doesn't stay still. It moves in different directions inside the body, like gentle winds that help everything work smoothly."

Tara tilted her head. "Winds? Inside our body?"

Uncle Vivek chuckled. "Yes! Not real air, but energy winds. Yogis say there are five main

ones, called the five vāyus. Each one has a special job."

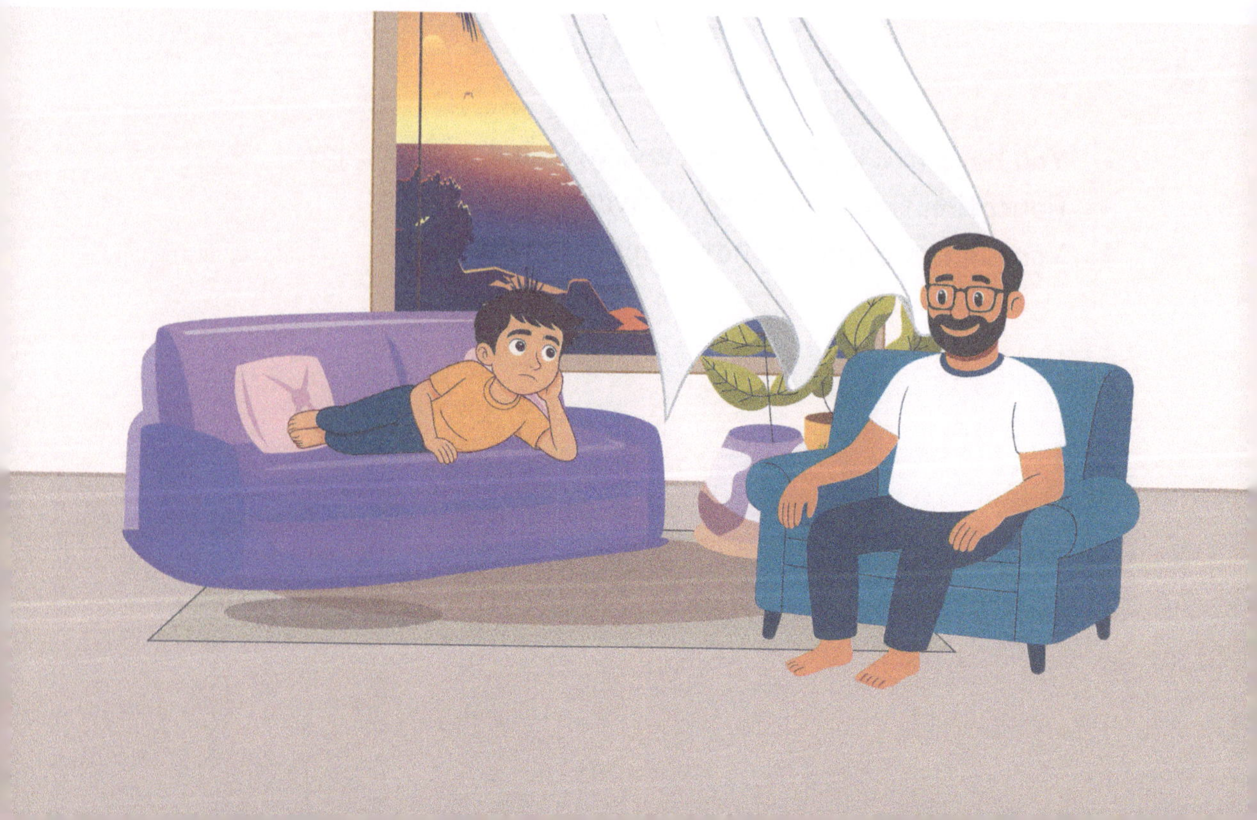

Meet Your Five Inner Winds

1. Prāna Vāyu - The Upward Energy

Lives in the chest. It powers your lungs and heart and helps you breathe in and feel full of life. Like the wind that lifts a kite high in the sky.

2. Apāna Vāyu - The Downward Energy

Apana vayu is located in the lower abdomen and pelvic region, specifically in the area from the navel to the perineum, governing elimination and supporting grounding/stability.

3. Samāna Vāyu - The Balancing Energy

Lives in the belly. It digests food and turns it into energy. Like a warm campfire that cooks your meal and keeps you glowing.

4. Udāna Vāyu - The Rising Energy

Lives in the throat and head. It helps you speak clearly and express your thoughts. Like air carrying your voice when you sing or speak with confidence.

5. Vyāna Vāyu - The Spreading Energy

Flows everywhere. It connects all the other winds and keeps blood, breath, and energy moving through your whole body. Like a gentle breeze spreading warmth from head to toe.

Everyday Examples

- Eating lunch — Samāna works.
- Running in sports — Vyāna spreads energy.
- Speaking in class — Udāna gives confidence.
- Breathing calmly — Prāna fills your lungs.
- Using the restroom — Apāna does its job.

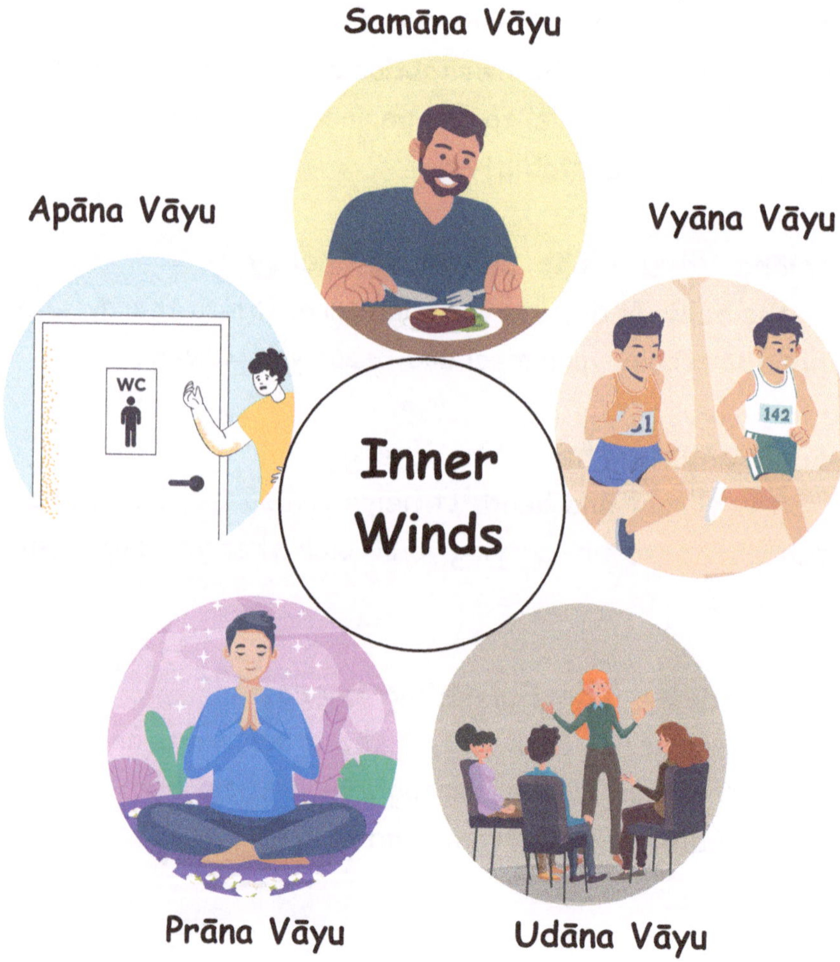

Science Connection

"These inner winds are another way of describing how our body works," explained Uncle Vivek.

Yogic Energy (Vāyu)	Body System	Main Function
Prāna	Breathing System	Inhale, heart rhythm
Samāna	Digestive System	Turns food into energy
Vyāna	Circulatory System	Blood and energy flow
Udāna	Nervous System & Speech	Voice, learning, expression
Apāna	Excretory System	Cleansing and release

"Ancient Yogis named these vāyus thousands of years ago to describe how life energy moves. Science today uses body systems and organs — both are ways of seeing the same amazing design inside us." When your inner winds move freely, you feel light, peaceful, and full of energy — ready to follow the call of life's breeze, wherever it leads.

Try This!

Feel the Five Energies

1. Prāna - Take a deep breath and feel your chest rise.
2. Apāna - Exhale slowly and imagine the air moving down to your feet.
3. Samāna - Place your hands on your belly after eating; feel the warmth of digestion.
4. Udāna - Say your name clearly and proudly; feel the energy rise through your throat.
5. Vyāna - Stretch your arms wide and feel your heartbeat spreading everywhere.

Takeaway

» The five inner winds (pañca-vāyu) keep your body and mind alive and balanced.

» They match what science calls the systems of breathing, digestion, and circulation.

» Yoga helps these winds flow freely — like a gentle breeze within you.

15. Chakras and the Spine

"Even miracles take a little time."
– Cinderella

Ravi lay flat on his mat, frowning. "Uncle, sometimes my chest feels heavy when I'm sad, or my stomach twists before an exam. Is that normal?"

"Yes," said Uncle Vivek. "Those feelings are connected to chakras—energy centers along your spine. Think of them like glowing wheels that spin energy in your body."

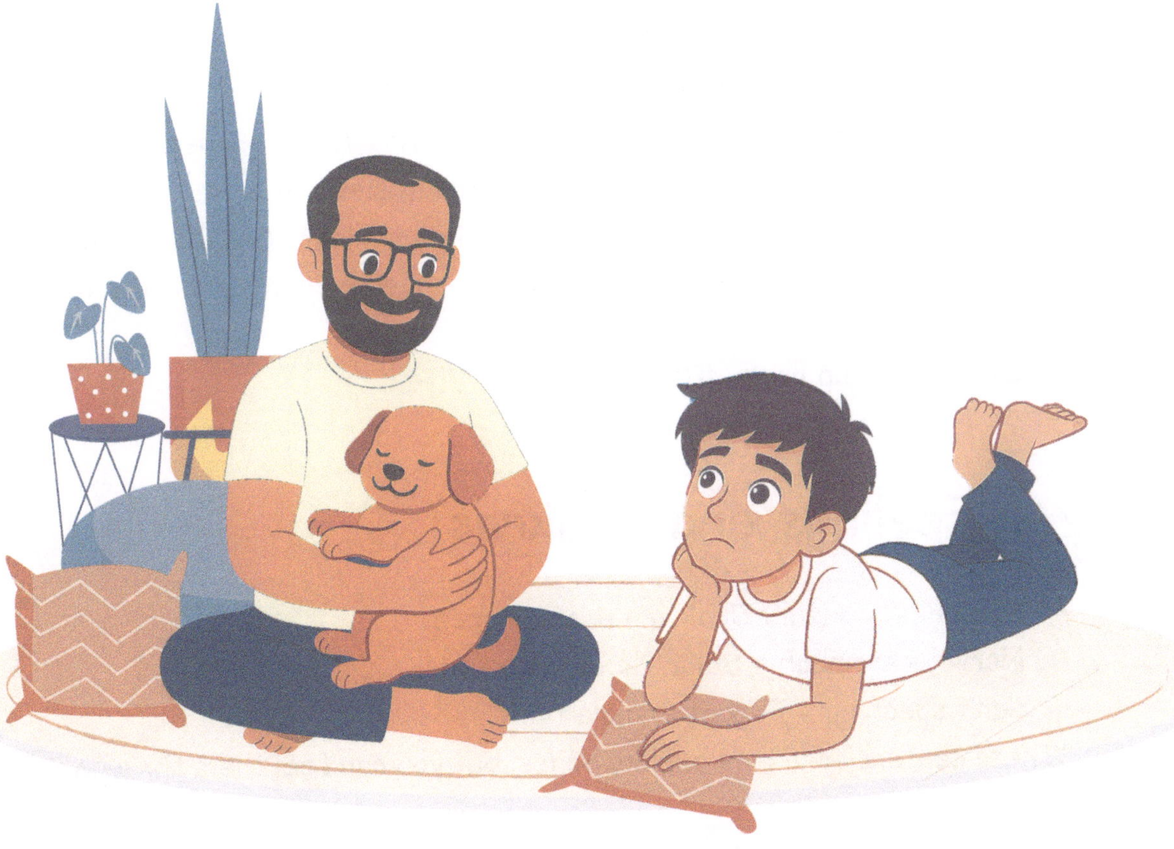

The Seven Chakras (Simplified for Kids)

Uncle Vivek traced his spine:

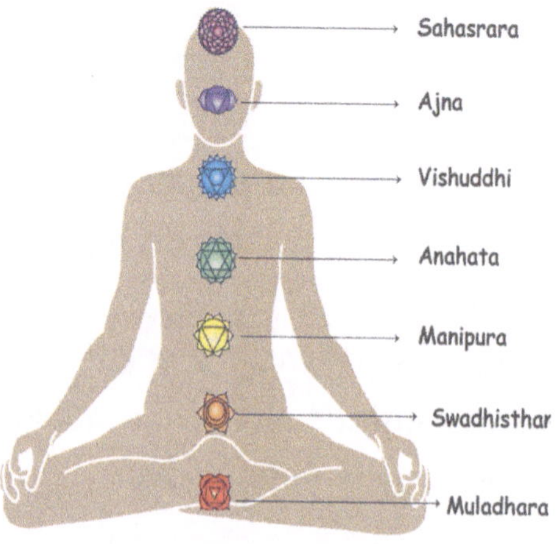

1. **Root Chakra (Muladhara)** - base of spine — safety, like tree roots.
2. **Sacral Chakra (Swadhisthana)** - lower belly — creativity and joy.
3. **Solar Plexus (Manipura)** - stomach area — courage and confidence.
4. **Heart Chakra (Anahata)** - chest — love and kindness.
5. **Throat Chakra (Vishuddhi)** - throat — clear speech, truth.
6. **Third Eye (Ajna)** - forehead — wisdom and intuition.
7. **Crown Chakra (Sahasrara)** - top of the head — peace and awareness, like a thousand-petaled lotus opening to light.

Tara nodded. "So, my chest heaviness is like my Heart Chakra feeling stressed, and Ravi's exam tummy is like his Solar Plexus reacting to worry?"

"You're picking up really fast!" said Uncle Vivek.

Feelings and Chakras

- Sad chest = Heart Chakra out of balance.
- Nervous stomach = Solar Plexus reacting.
- Can't speak up = Throat Chakra tight.

"These centers aren't visible like bones, but you can feel them through emotions."

The Power of Sound - Om

"Some people ask why Yogis chant," Ravi said.

"Because sound helps balance energy," Uncle Vivek replied. "The most common sound is Om (Aum)."

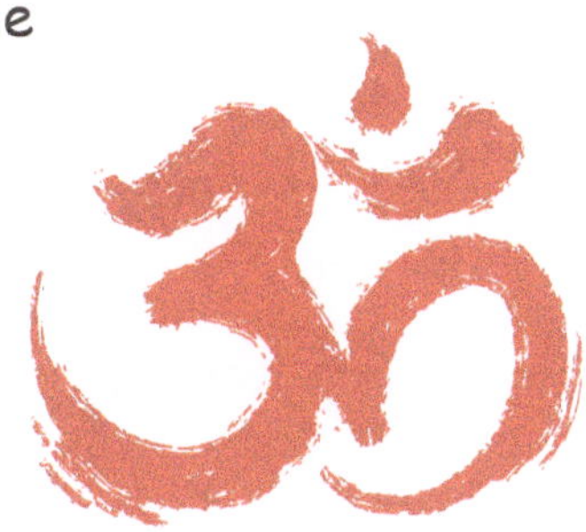

- "A" starts in the belly.
- "U" moves through the chest.
- "M" ends in the head.

"After the sound, silence follows—and that silence is powerful too."

Science Connection

"Scientists explain chakras in modern terms too," Uncle Vivek said. "The solar plexus has nerve bundles that react to stress. The heart links emotions and heartbeat. The throat connects to speech. Chakras are like poetic maps for the same body-mind links."

"Chakras are like Wi-Fi signals, aren't they?" Ravi joked. "You can't see them, but you feel them."

"Now I understand better!" said Tara.

Try This!

Spine Breathing

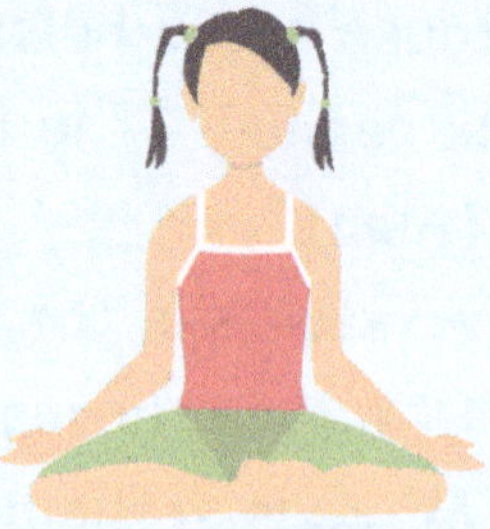

1. Sit tall.
2. Inhale — imagine energy rising up the spine.
3. Exhale — imagine it flowing back down.

Heart Opener

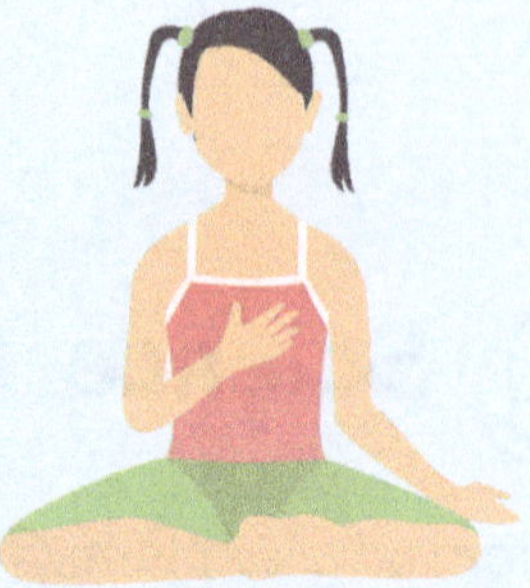

1. Place hand on chest.
2. Inhale — picture sunlight filling your chest.
3. Exhale — imagine sharing kindness.

Voice Flow

1. Say "Aaa" from belly.
2. Say "Uuu" from chest.
3. Say "Mmm" buzzing in your head.

Takeaway

» Chakras = Seven energy buttons along your spine.
» Each links to feelings, thoughts, and health.
» Om = full-body sound + silence that calms.
» Yoga balances your inner "energy Wi-Fi."

Gratitude Journaling

Take a moment to introspect!

My strengths are...

I want to improve on...

16. Yoga and Science - Wisdom Meets Discovery

"The important thing is to never stop questioning."
- Albert Einstein

Rain tapped on the window as Ravi balanced a pencil on his lip. "Uncle, Yoga feels ancient. But do scientists even care about it today?"

"Good question," Uncle Vivek said. "For centuries, sages explored Yoga in forests. Now scientists study it in labs and hospitals. And guess what? Much of what they find matches what Yogis knew long ago."

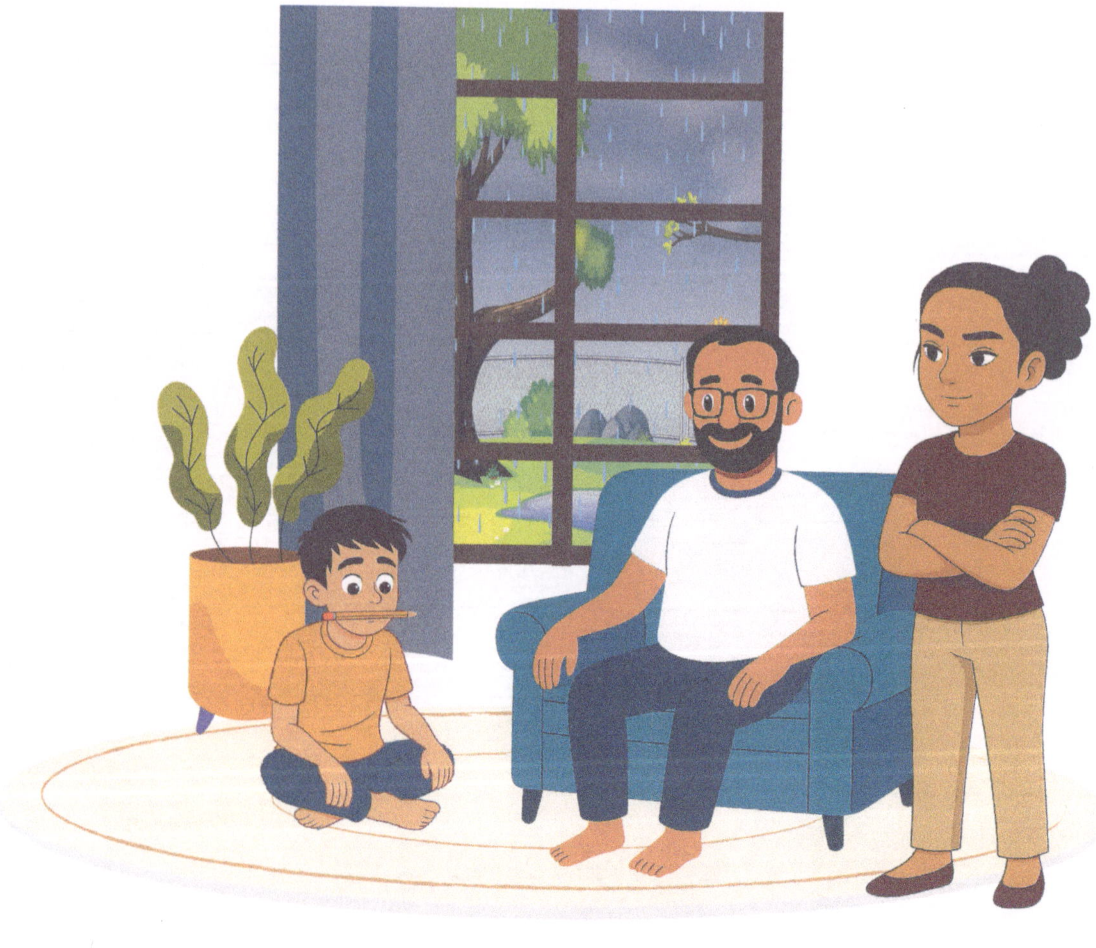

Your Brain on Yoga

"At Harvard, Scientists found that just 8 weeks of Yoga or meditation increased grey matter in memory and focus areas of the brain. Stress areas became quieter."

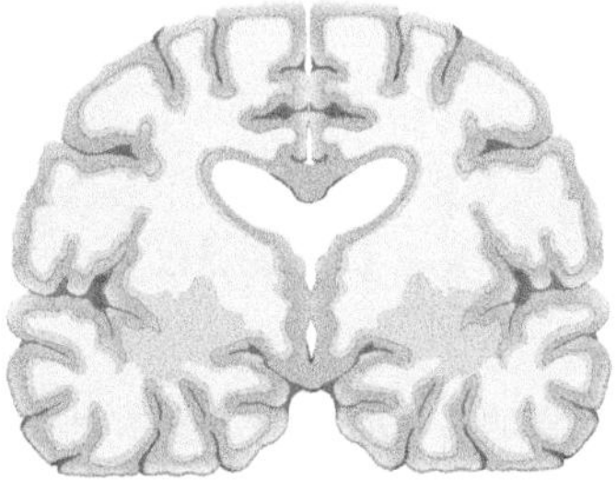

"Whoa," Ravi said. "Uncle, so is Yoga like brain training?" "Yes, like a gym for your brain!" Uncle Vivek laughed.

For Heart and Emotions

"Yoga also improves heart rate variability (HRV)—a sign of a flexible, calm heart. It balances emotions by boosting happy hormones and lowering stress ones."

Tara placed her hand on her chest. "I have noticed that after performing Yoga, my heart feels calmer, and my mood becomes lighter."

"Yes, even I feel stronger and full of energy." said Ravi.

Growth and Development

Ravi held an old photo. "Uncle, I was so small!"

"That is growth," Uncle Vivek said. "Your body becomes taller and stronger. You can measure it."

Tara asked, "Then what is development?"

"Development is what happens inside — clearer thinking, better focus, calmer feelings, wiser choices. You cannot measure it with a ruler."

Ravi nodded. "So growth is outside, development is inside."
"Exactly," Uncle Vivek said. "Yoga helps both growth and development. It keeps the body healthy and the mind steady."

Nobel Minds & Yoga

"Even Nobel Prize research shows Yoga slows aging," Vivek explained. "Elizabeth Blackburn discovered that stress shrinks protective caps on DNA, called telomeres. Yoga helps keep them longer, so your cells stay healthier."

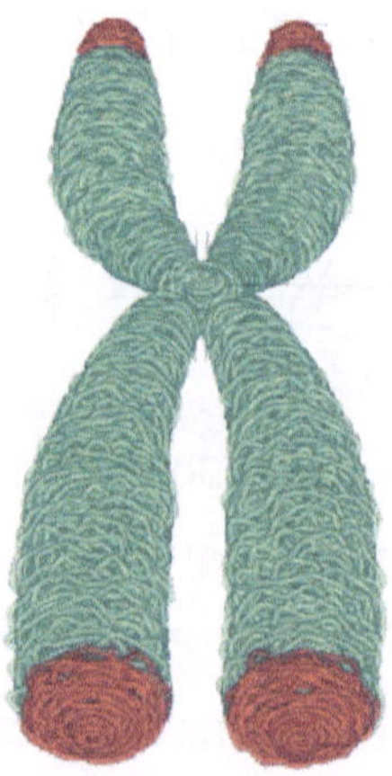

"Wow! That's like an anti-aging shield!" Ravi exclaimed.
Uncle Vivek added, "Some Nobel winners respect Yoga too. John Eccles studied the brain and said Yoga helps self-awareness. Brian Josephson believed meditation connects science and consciousness. Even leaders used it for calm decision-making."
"So, Yoga works in classrooms and countries?" Tara laughed. "Exactly, dear Tara," he smiled.

Research Around the World

Yoga is studied at Harvard, MIT, Stanford, Oxford, AIIMS, NIMHANS, and even NASA (to help astronauts manage stress in space!).
"Space Yoga?" Ravi shouted.
"Yes," Uncle Vivek chuckled. "Breathing keeps astronauts calm too."

Pioneers of Scientific Yoga

"It all began with pioneers like Swami Kuvalyanand, who studied Yoga with scientific tools in the 1920s. Later, teachers like B.K.S. Iyengar and Maharshi Mahesh Yogi made Yoga famous worldwide. They showed it helps daily life, health, and healing."

Try This!

Yoga Science Experiment

1. Do 5 slow breaths.
2. Notice your heart beat.
3. Write or draw how you feel.
4. Compare with how you felt before.

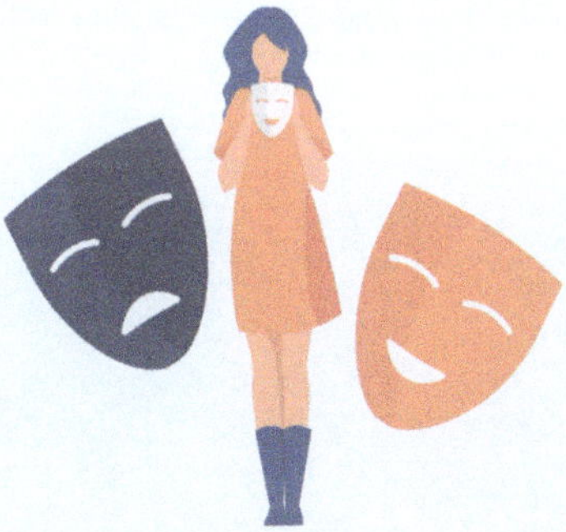

Takeaway

» Ancient wisdom + modern science = same truths.
» Yoga strengthens brain, heart, emotions, even DNA health.
» Even astronauts and Nobel scientists value Yoga.
» Every time you practice, you're joining the world's biggest science experiment.

Part V
Adventure & Beyond

"With great power comes great responsibility."
- Spider-Man

Bring Yoga into your daily life with balance, play, and care

Yoga isn't only on a mat—it's a way to live. From morning to night, online and offline, you can use Yoga to stay balanced, safe, and joyful.

In this part, Ravi and Tara learn:

- How to build daily routines
- How to balance screens with "green time"
- How to make Yoga a game, journal, or experiment
- How to practice safely with patience and care

17. Build Your Daily Routine - Mornings to Nights

"I meditate, do yoga, and have good people around you that you can trust."
— Jennie, Blackpink

One morning, Ravi stumbled out of bed with messy hair.

"Why does waking up feel harder than math homework?" he groaned.

Tara was already stretching on her mat. "Because you don't have a routine," she teased.

Uncle Vivek smiled. "She's right. Yoga isn't only poses. It's also about daily rhythms—how you wake up, move, eat, and rest. A good routine keeps your body, mind, and energy balanced all day."

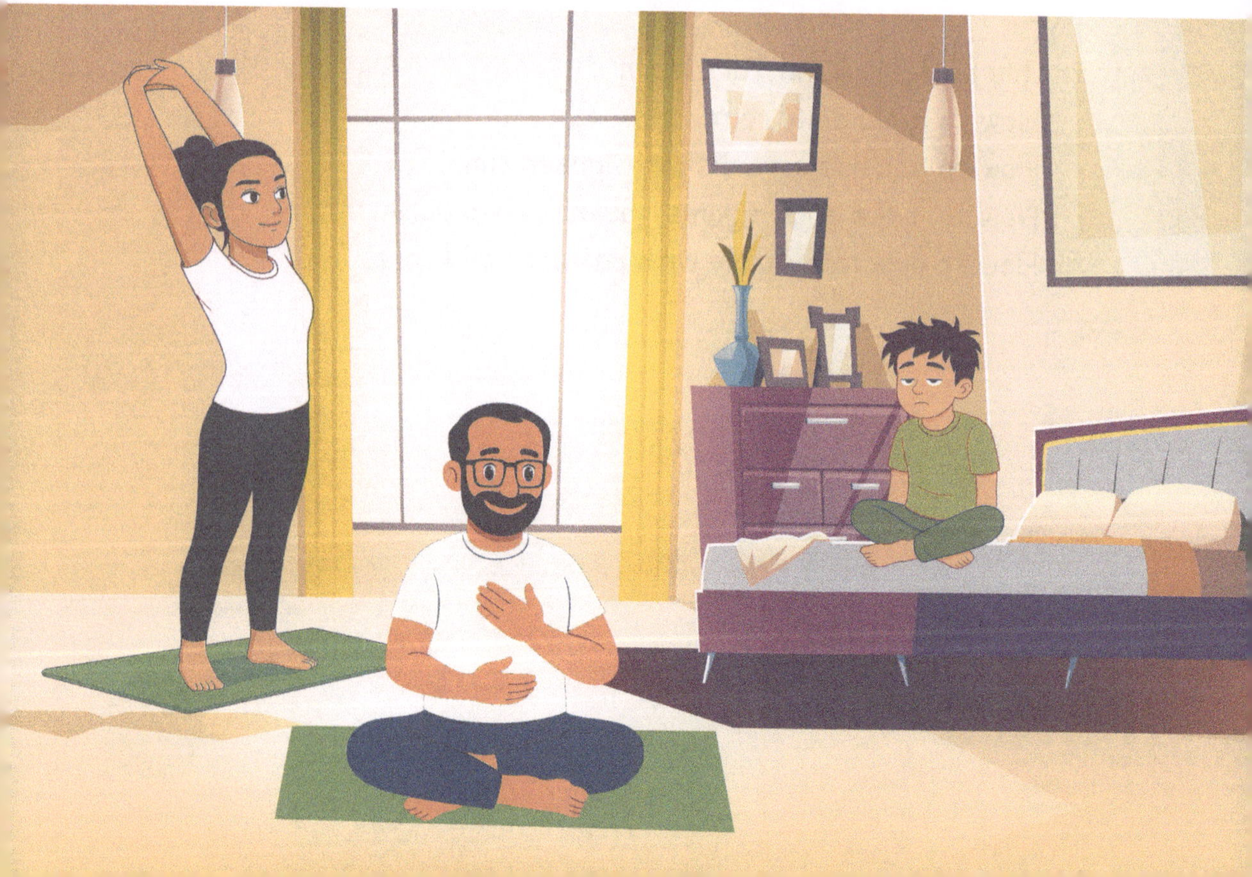

Food and Mood - The Three Gunas

"Every food carries a mood," Vivek explained.

- **Sattva foods** - fresh fruits, veggies, nuts, milk — calm, happy, clear.
- **Rajas foods** - spicy, sugary, cola — restless, jumpy.
- **Tamas foods** - stale, greasy, junk — lazy, sleepy.

"Meaning if I want superhero energy, I should eat more Sattva foods?" Tara asked. "Yes! Let's begin right away." Uncle Vivek nodded.

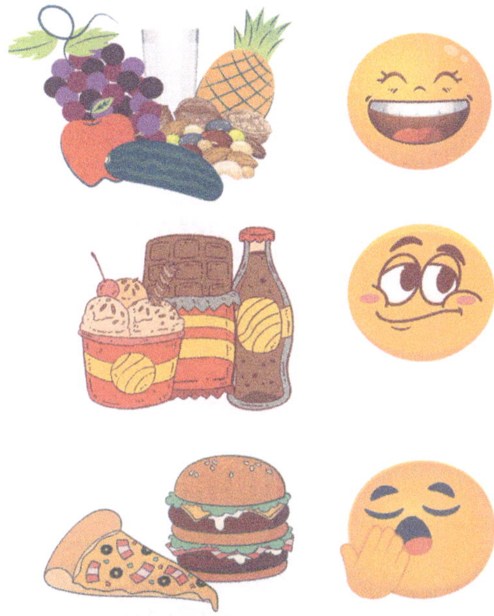

Morning: Start with Awareness

"Most people wake up and grab their phone," said Vivek. "But how you start shapes your day."

3 simple habits:

1. One minute of quiet breathing
2. Gentle stretches - Cat-Cow or Forward Fold
3. Gratitude thought - name one thing you're glad for

Midday: Recharge Instead of Crash

"By lunchtime, you may feel tired," Uncle Vivek said. "Instead of eating sugar- rich foods like chocolates or scrolling, try resetting with movement and breath."

Quick 2-minute reset:

- Roll shoulders back
- Take 5 belly breaths
- Do 1 standing pose (Tree, Triangle, or Warrior)
- Drink water

Evening: Let Go of the Day

In the evening, Tara sometimes felt overloaded.

"Yoga adds a pause," Vivek said. "Stretch gently, journal one reflection, or sit for a few breaths."

Night: Prepare for Rest

"Rest isn't lazy," Uncle Vivek reminded them. "It's repair time for body and brain."

Tips for bedtime:

- Turn off screens 30 min earlier
- Try Legs-Up-the-Wall Pose for 5 min
- Inhale for 4 counts, exhale for 4
- Whisper one kind thought to yourself
- Chant Om 11 times for peaceful sleep

Try This!

Routine Map

1. Fold paper into 4 boxes: Morning, Midday, Evening, Night. Draw or write one small Yoga habit in each.
2. Try for 1 week and notice your energy.

Takeaway

» Routines shape energy from morning to night.

» Food affects mood—choose wisely.

» Small pauses = big resets.

» Rest and sleep are part of Yoga too.

Gratitude Journaling

Take a moment to make a creative drawing about the magical moments that make you happy!
I feel happy when...

18. Yoga in a Digital World - Lessons from Screen-Time Heroes

"Don't be trapped in someone else's dream."
– RM, K-pop band BTS

"Be honest," Tara said, raising an eyebrow. "How many hours did you spend on screen-time today?"

Ravi looked sheepish. "Umm... for school or for fun?"

"Both count," Tara replied.

"You're not alone," Uncle Vivek said kindly. "We all live in a digital world now. But Yoga can help us use screens wisely."

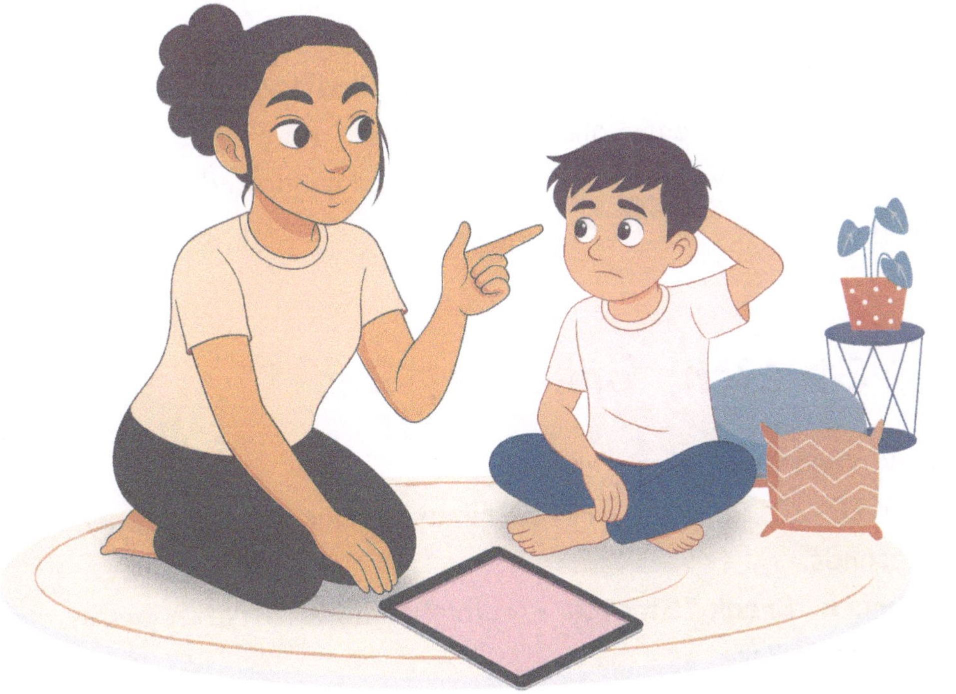

Screens Are Not the Enemy

"Screens aren't bad," Vivek explained. "They help us learn, play, and connect. But too much screen-time without awareness causes problems."

Too much screen time can:

- Dry your eyes
- Weaken posture
- Shorten attention span
- Disturb sleep
- Drain mood and energy

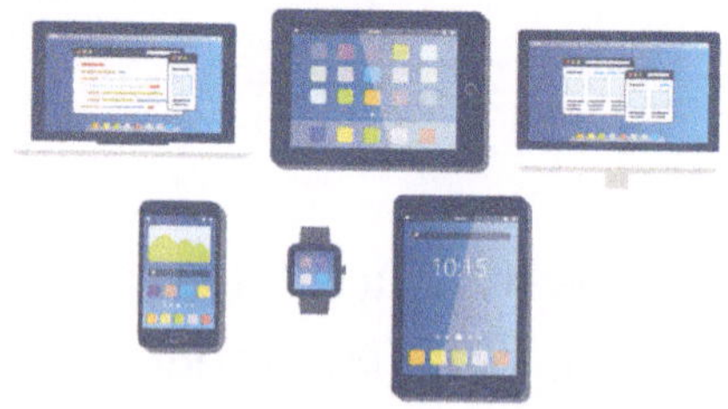

"Yoga isn't about throwing devices away. It's about noticing when tech helps you—and when it starts using you."

Know Your Signals

Tara nodded. "I can tell when I've scrolled too long—my shoulders ache, my head feels heavy, and I lose track of time.

"Exactly," Uncle Vivek said. "Your body and mind send signals when it's too much."

Stretch, Breathe, Reset

Simple Yoga tips for screen life:

- **20-20-20 Rule** - every 20 minutes, look 20 feet away for 20 seconds.
- **Screen Break Stretch** - roll shoulders, stretch arms, or do Mountain Pose.

- **Mindful Scrolling** - ask before opening an app: "Why am I here? What do I want to feel?"
- **Bedtime Tech-Off** - turn off screens 30-60 minutes before bed.
- **Green Time for Screen Time** - for every hour online, add time outdoors.

Screen-Time Heroes

"Even famous people use Yoga to stay balanced," Vivek added.

- Lionel Messi - stretches for focus and flexibility
- Emma Watson - meditation for calm
- Virat Kohli - Yoga for focus and discipline
- Alia Bhatt - daily Yoga to recharge
- J.K. Rowling - breath and quiet for creativity

"And Kung Fu Panda reminds us: inner peace is the real superpower!"

Tara's Tip: Make Tech Your Tool

"I made a Yoga folder on my tablet," Tara said proudly. "It has calming music, a timer, my favorite Yoga videos, and a gratitude journal app. I didn't delete games—I just added balance."

Ravi nodded. "Okay, I'll add a stretch after every game level."

Try This!

Upgrade Your Tech Habit

Pick one upgrade this week:

- No phone at dining table
- Stretch after every game level
- Tech-free mornings

Takeaway

» Screens can help or hurt—it depends how you use them.

» Notice your body's warning signs.

» Balance screen time with green time.

» Tech should be your tool, not your boss.

19. Ask, Play, Reflect - Games, Journals, and Experiments

"Every child is an artist."
- Picasso

One evening, while watching a video of people practicing Yoga in different countries, Ravi asked, "I know Yoga began in India, but is it celebrated only here?"

Tara smiled. "Not really! The United Nations saw how people everywhere were enjoying Yoga and declared 21 June as International Yoga Day, so the whole world could celebrate it together."

Uncle Vivek nodded. "That's right! The International Yoga Day, with people from more than 190 countries joining at the same time — a true gift from India to the world."

Ravi's eyes lit up. "That's amazing! When we practice Yoga, we're part of something global — all breathing together."

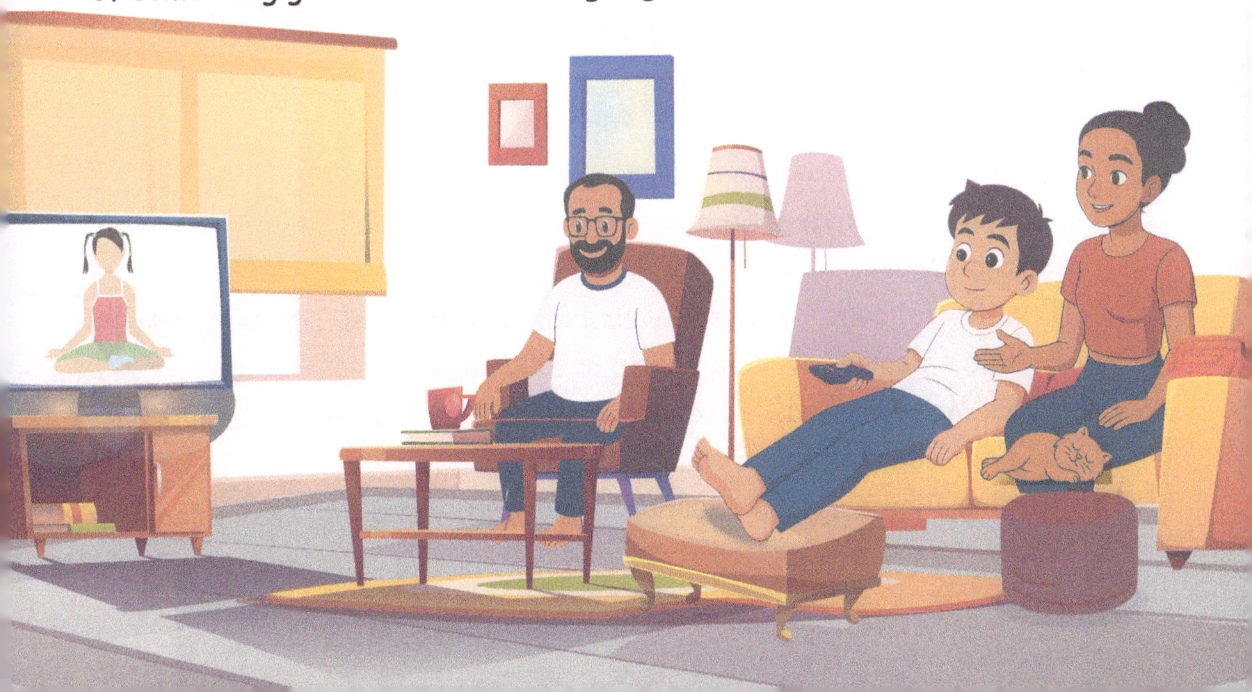

He then flopped onto his mat and sighed. "I like Yoga," he said, "but sometimes I get bored doing the same poses again."

Tara laughed. "Then let's make it a game!"

"Can I invent my own pose?" Ravi asked eagerly.

"You can invent your whole practice," said Uncle Vivek with a smile. "Yoga isn't about rules — it's about discovery."

Yoga as Play

Yoga doesn't have to be serious. It can be playful, like a treasure hunt or puzzle. Yoga can be:

- A game of balance
- A challenge of focus
- A flow that matches your mood
- A puzzle where you discover what works for you

Try These Games

- **Pose Charades** - Act out a Yoga pose without naming it. Others guess. Bonus: add animal sounds!
- **Balance Challenge** - Who can hold Tree Pose the longest? Try with eyes closed.
- **Breath Balloons** - Pretend your belly is a balloon. Inhale = inflate, exhale = float away. Add colors or silly names.
- **Yoga Memory Trail** - Make a sequence of 3-5 poses. Repeat and add one new pose each round.
- **Feeling Flow** - Pick a feeling (happy, sad, sleepy, brave). Create a short Yoga sequence for it.

Asking Questions

"Yoga is also about curiosity," Uncle Vivek said. "Not just doing, but asking." Sample journal questions:

- What made me smile today?
- Where do I feel strong in my body?
- What helped me calm down?
- How did my breath feel this morning?
- Who needs kindness from me today?

Journals & Experiments

"You can write, doodle, or record voice notes," Tara suggested. "Yoga is also a lab," Uncle Vivek added. "You can experiment."

Examples:

- What happens if I breathe slower when angry?
- Does stretching in the morning help me focus in class?
- What if I sit still for 1 minute before eating?
- What changes if I speak kindly all day?

"You are the scientist," Uncle Vivek said.

Try This!

1. Invent a new pose and give it a name.
2. Write or draw one moment when you used Yoga off the mat.
3. Track how you feel before and after 5 slow breaths.
4. Create a comic strip of your Yoga day.

Guess the Pose!

Now try demonstrating various poses and make your friends guess the pose!

Takeaway

» Yoga = play, discovery, and reflection.
» Games, journals, and experiments make practice fun.
» You are both the player and the scientist.

20. Safety First - Precautions for Young Yogis

"Luck favors the prepared."
- Edna Mode, The Incredibles

One afternoon, Ravi tried a headstand he had seen on YouTube. He kicked up—then toppled sideways and hit the floor with a thud.

"Ow!" he groaned, holding his shoulder.

Tara rushed over. "Ravi! Who told you to do that?"

"No one," he muttered. "It just looked cool."

Uncle Vivek gently helped him sit up. "And now your shoulder is telling you a different story. Yoga is not about stunts. It is about listening to your body."

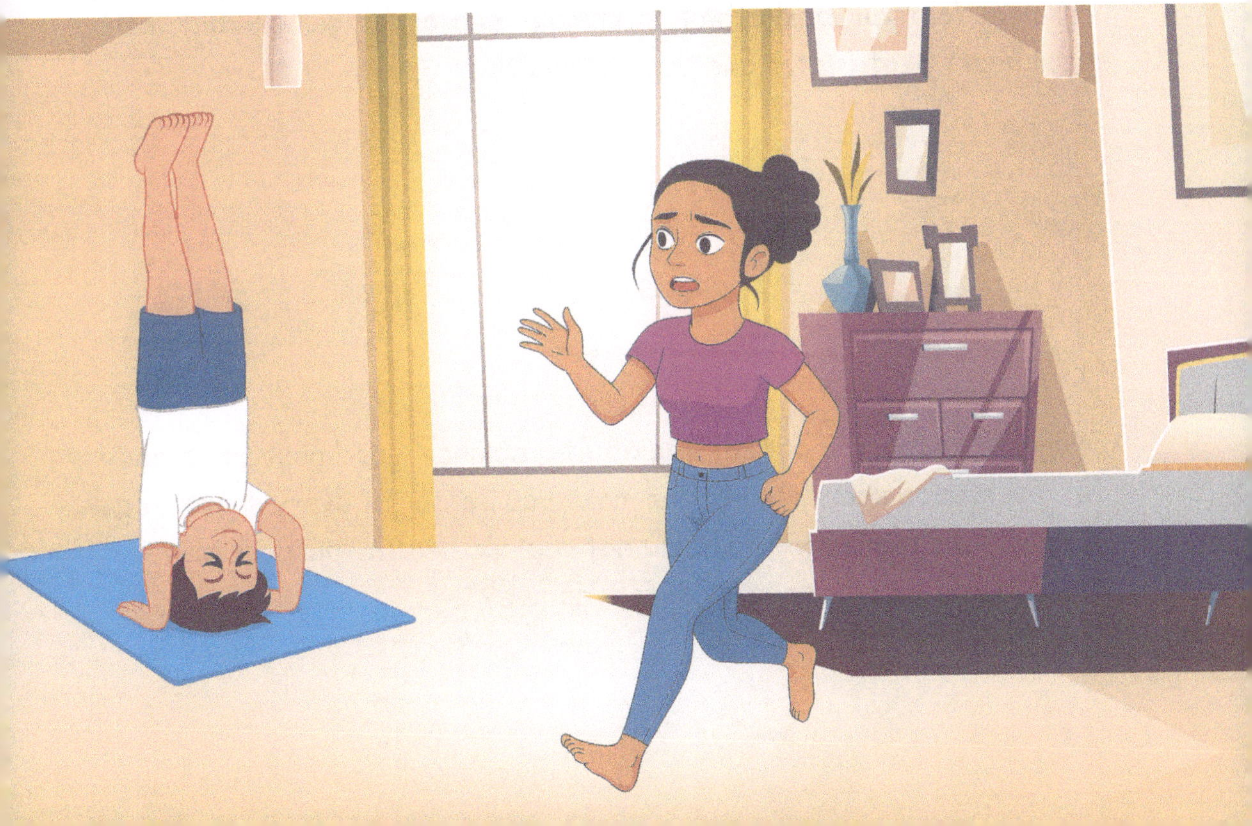

Yoga Is Not a Competition

"It's easy to get excited," Uncle Vivek said. "But the strongest Yogis are not the ones who bend the farthest or balance the longest. The real strength is knowing your limits."

Tara nodded. "I once skipped warm-up and pulled a muscle. Now I always start simple." Uncle Vivek smiled. "Exactly. Yoga teaches patience as much as it teaches posture."

Growing Up with Yoga

"Since you both are still growing," Uncle Vivek said, "Yoga must be practiced wisely. Up to the age of twelve, your bones and muscles are changing very fast. Yoga alone is not enough for balanced growth."

He continued, "It works best when combined with outdoor sports—running, football, basketball, swimming, and other games that make your heart beat faster and build strength."

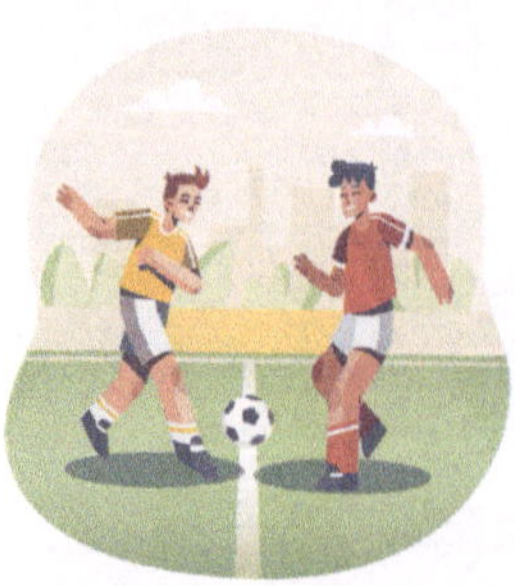

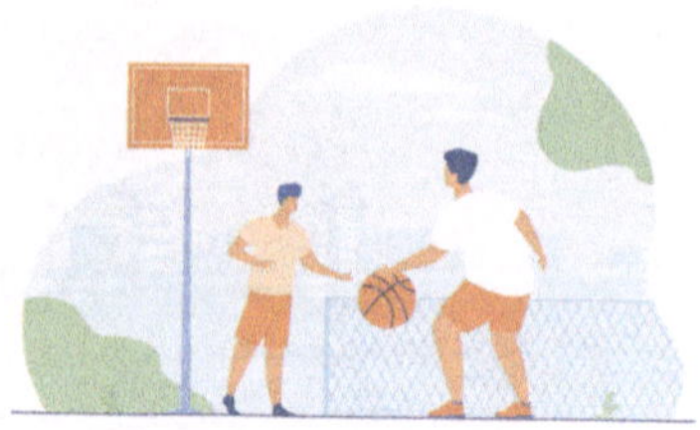

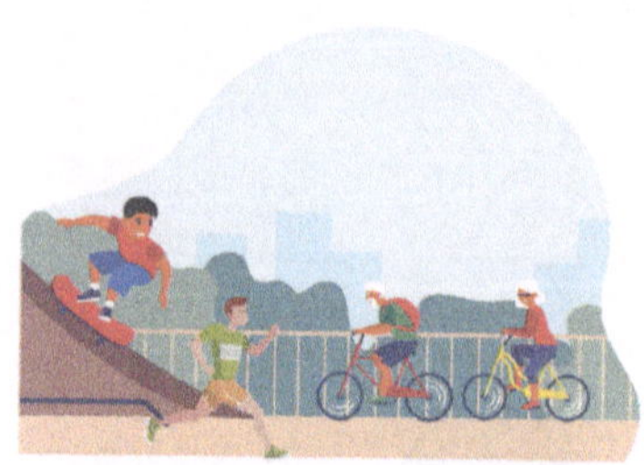

"Yoga helps too," he added. "Flexibility, balance, good posture, steady breathing, and short meditation make you better at every sport. Yoga supports your growth—it should not replace healthy outdoor play."

Ravi asked, "So what can we safely do now?"

"At this age," Uncle Vivek replied, "you can enjoy fast-paced Suryanamaskars, simple Pranayama, and short meditation or relaxation. Hard or long-held postures can wait for later."

"And remember," he said firmly, "always practice Yoga and sports under trained experts. Guidance keeps you safe."

Golden Rules for Young Buddies

Uncle Vivek shared his list of safety tips:

- Learn with a teacher - Always practice under a trained Yoga instructor.
- Start simple - Master basics first.
- Warm up - Always prepare your muscles.
- Never force a pose - Pain means stop.
- Use a safe space - A mat or carpet, never slippery floors.
- Breathe steadily - If your breath feels shaky, slow down and relax.
- No headstands alone - Inversions only with an expert.
- Protect your neck and spine - Move gently.
- Rest when needed - Yoga is not a race.
- End with meditation or relaxation - A calm mind makes Yoga complete.

Bodies Change Every Day

"What felt easy yesterday might feel stiff today," Uncle Vivek reminded them. "That's normal. Respect your body's changes."

Tara added, "And don't compare with others. Everyone grows differently."

CLOSING THE CIRCLE

Ravi lay back in Savasana, smiling. "Lesson learned—no superhero stunts without training."

Tara laughed. "And no skipping warm-ups."

Uncle Vivek placed a gentle hand on their shoulders. "Good. Yoga is not about how much you can do, but how you do it with patience, kindness, and care."

Yoga teaches us to care for our body, calm our mind, and choose wisely—every day.

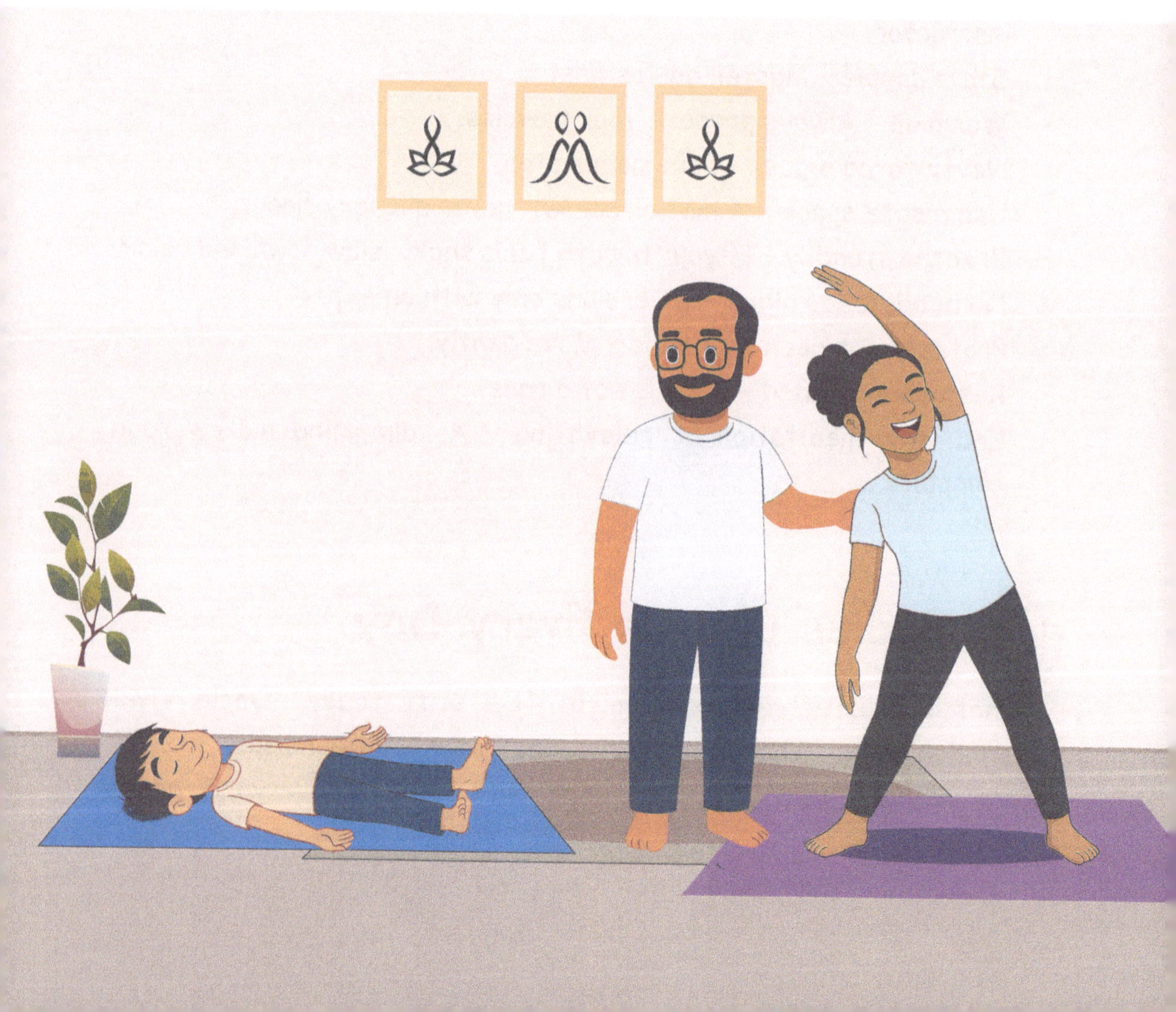

Try This!

Safety Check

Before practice, pause and ask:

1. Have I warmed up?
2. Are you hydrated enough?
3. Is my space clear and safe?
4. Am I doing this to feel good—or just to impress?

Takeaway

- Yoga is about awareness and care—not stunts or competition.
- Safe practice keeps Yoga joyful, steady, and lifelong.
- Listen to your body today—it grows, changes, and needs respect.
- Yoga works best when guided by teachers and balanced with outdoor play.

Glossary

Words You Would Love to Know!

"Yoga is an art, a science, and a philosophy."
— B.K.S. Iyengar

A

- **Adiyogi (आदियोगी)** - "The first yogi," another name for Shiva, said to have shared Yoga with the earliest seekers.
- **Adrenaline** - A "rush" hormone your body makes during stress or excitement; it makes your heart beat faster and muscles ready to move.
- **ADHD (Attention Deficit Hyperactivity Disorder)** - A condition where kids may find it hard to sit still, focus, or control impulses; Yoga and breathing can sometimes help calm the mind.
- **Ahimsa (अहिंसा)** - Non-harming; being kind in thoughts, words, and actions.
- **Alveoli** - Tiny air sacs in your lungs where oxygen passes into the blood.
- **Annamaya Kosha (अन्नमय कोश)** - The physical body layer, made of food and matter.
- **Anāhata (अनाहत)** - The heart chakra, linked with love and kindness.
- **Āsana (आसन)** - A Yoga posture or pose, like Tree Pose or Cobra.
- **Ājñā (आज्ञा)** - The "third eye" chakra, between your eyebrows, linked with wisdom and clarity.
- **Anxiety** - A feeling of worry or nervousness that doesn't go away easily.
- **Awareness** - Noticing what is happening in the present moment — in your body, breath, mind, or surroundings. Awareness is the first step in Yoga.

B

- **Balasana (बालासन)** - Child's Pose, a resting position where you fold forward with knees bent.
- **Bhakti Yoga (भक्तियोग)** - The Yoga of love and devotion, like singing, prayer, or gratitude. Brain grey matter - The part of your brain that helps with memory, focus, and learning.

C

- **Camel Pose (Ustrasana)** - A backbend Yoga pose that opens your chest and stretches your spine.
- **Chakra (चक्र)** - Means "wheel." Energy centers in your body that affect feelings, thoughts, and health.
- **Citta (चित्त)** - The mind; includes thoughts, emotions, and memory.
- **Circulatory system** - The body system that pumps blood through your heart and blood vessels.
- **Consciousness** - Your inner awareness — the part of you that knows "I am." It's more than thoughts or feelings. Consciousness is like a light inside that helps you notice your body, breath, mind, and the world around you. In Yoga, it means being awake not just with open eyes, but also awake inside.
- **Cortisol** - A stress hormone your body makes when you feel pressure or fear.

D

- **Diaphragm** - A dome-shaped muscle under your lungs that helps you breathe deeply.
- **Dharana (धारणा)** - Concentration; focusing your mind on one thing.
- **Dhyāna (ध्यान)** - Meditation; quiet awareness without distraction.

- **DNA (Deoxyribonucleic Acid)** - The "instruction book" inside every cell that tells it how to work.
- **Dopamine** - A "reward" chemical in the brain that makes you feel excited or motivated.

E

- **Endorphins** - Chemicals in your brain that make you feel happy and relaxed.
- **Energy centers** - Another way to describe chakras, places where body and mind connect.

F

- **Focus / Concentration** - The ability to pay attention to one thing without being distracted.

G

- **Guna (गुण)** - In Yoga philosophy, gunas are the three natural qualities or moods that shape how we feel and act. Sattva - calm, clear, and balanced (like sunshine after rain). Rajas - active, busy, and restless (like a racing car). Tamas - heavy, dull, or sleepy (like a foggy morning). These three qualities are always present in different amounts. Yoga helps increase sattva — the peaceful and happy state — so our body, mind, and actions stay in harmony.

H

- **Hatha Yoga (हठ योग)** - A traditional style of Yoga with balanced poses and breathing.

- **Heart Rate Variability (HRV)** - Tiny changes between heartbeats; shows how flexible and healthy your heart is.
- **Hormones** - Chemical messengers in your body that affect growth, mood, and energy.

I

- **Ida (इडा)** - A main energy channel in Yoga, linked with calmness and creativity.
- **Immune system** - Your body's defense team that fights germs and keeps you healthy.
- **Iyengar Yoga** - A Yoga style that uses props (blocks, straps) and focuses on alignment.

J

- **Jñāna Yoga (ज्ञान योग)** - The Yoga of knowledge and wisdom.

K

- **Karma Yoga (कर्म योग)** - The Yoga of action and service, helping others.
- **Koshas (कोश)** - The five "layers" of a human being: body, energy, mind, wisdom, and joy.
- **Kundalini (कुण्डलिनी)** - Described as coiled energy at the base of the spine that rises through practice.

L

- **Lungs** - Organs that bring oxygen into your body and release carbon dioxide.

M

- **Mandala (मण्डल)** - A circle design used for focus, meditation, and creativity.
- **Manomaya Kosha (मनोमय कोश)** - The mental-emotional layer, where thoughts and feelings live.
- **Mantra (मंत्र)** - A special word or sound repeated for focus, like Om.
- **Meditation** - Sitting quietly to focus your mind and calm your thoughts.
- **Metabolism** - The process by which your body turns food into energy.
- **Microbes** - Tiny living things (like bacteria) that live in your gut and help digestion.
- **Muladhara (मूलाधार)** - The root chakra, at the base of the spine, linked with safety and strength.

N

- **NASA (National Aeronautics and Space Administration)** - The U.S. space agency that studies astronauts, planets, and even breathing in space.
- **Nadis (नाडि)** - Energy pathways in the body where life-energy (prana) flows.
- **Nervous system** - The network of nerves and the brain that controls body and mind signals. Neurotransmitters - Brain chemicals (like serotonin and dopamine) that carry messages and affect mood.
- **Niyama (नियम)** - Personal habits in Yoga, like cleanliness, contentment, and self-study.

O

- **Ojus (ओजस्)** - In Yoga and Ayurveda, Ojus is your inner energy that gives strength,
- immunity, and glow. It is built from good food, rest, breath, and kind thoughts — the secret sparkle that keeps you healthy and happy.

P

- **Pancha Kosha (पंच कोश)** - The five sheaths or layers of being, from body to bliss.
- **Panchaprana (पंचप्राण)** - The five vital energy forces: prana, apana, samana, udana, vyana.
- **Patanjali (पंतजलि)** - Ancient sage who wrote the Yoga Sutras, organizing Yoga into clear steps.
- **Piṅgalā (पिंगला)** - An energy channel in Yoga, linked with action and heat.
- **Prana (प्राण)** - Life-energy, carried by breath through the body.
- **Pranayama (प्राणायाम)** - Breath practices that guide and control prana.
- **Pratyahara (प्रत्याहार)** - Turning attention inward, away from distractions.

Q

- **Qi** - In Chinese tradition, Qi means "life energy" or "vital force." It's the invisible energy that flows through all living things, keeping the body and mind active and balanced.

R

- **Ravi (रवि)** - A Sanskrit word meaning Sun. In Indian tradition, the sun represents energy, light, and life.
- **Restorative Yoga** - A slow Yoga style that uses props and long holds for relaxation.

S

- **Samadhi (समाधी)** - A state of peaceful union, feeling connected with everything.
- **Samana (समान)** - One of the five pranas; centered in the belly, helps digestion.
- **Samavrtti Pranayama (समवृत्ति् प्राणायाम)** - Equal breathing, inhaling and exhaling for the same count.
- **Sattva** - In Yoga philosophy, the quality of balance, clarity, and harmony.
- **Savasana (शवासन)** - Also called Corpse Pose. A resting pose where you lie flat on your back with eyes closed, arms and legs relaxed, and breathe slowly. It looks simple, but it's important because it helps the body rest, the mind settle, and consciousness become clear and calm.
- **Serotonin** - A "feel-good" chemical in the brain that helps mood, sleep, and calm.
- **Shat Chakra (षट्चक्र)** - The six main chakras, or spinning energy centers, along the spine.
- **Shiva (शिव)** - In Yoga tradition, the Adiyogi, the first yogi who shared the secrets of Yoga.
- **Spirituality** - Spirituality means looking inside yourself to find peace, kindness, and connection. It helps us live with love, care, and balance.

- **Stress hormones** - Chemicals (like adrenaline and cortisol) released when your body feels pressure.
- **Sushumna (सषुम्ना)** - The central energy channel along the spine.
- **Svadhisthana (स्वाधिष्ठान)** - The sacral chakra, below the navel, linked with creativity and joy.

T

- **Tara (तारा)** - A Sanskrit word meaning Star. Stars are symbols of guidance, hope, and direction, shining even in darkness.
- **Tree Pose (Vŕkśāsana / वृक्षासन)** - A balancing Yoga pose where you stand on one leg like a tree.

U

- **Udana (उदान)** - One of the five pranas; upward energy that helps with speech and confidence.
- **Ustrasana (ऊष्ट्रासन)** - Camel Pose, a chest-opening backbend.

V

- **Vagus nerve** - A long nerve that helps calm the body, lower stress, and improve digestion.
- **Vinyasa (विन्यास)** - A flowing style of Yoga where movement follows the breath.
- **Visuddhi (विशुद्धि)** - The throat chakra, linked with speaking truth and communication.
- **Vivek (विवेक)** - A Sanskrit word that means wisdom, clear thinking, and knowing the difference between what is right and what is not. In this book, Uncle Vivek is the wise friend who helps connect Yoga's ancient wisdom with modern science.

- **Vyana (व्यान)** - One of the five pranas; spreads energy throughout the body for circulation and
- movement.

X

- **X-ray** - A special kind of invisible light that can pass through the body to take pictures of bones and organs. Doctors use X-rays to see what's inside the body without surgery.

Y

- **Yoga (योग)** - From Sanskrit "yuj," meaning to join or unite and also to follow discipline —the practice of bringing body, breath, and mind together.
- **Yoga Sutras (योग सूत्र)** - A collection of best practices of Yoga by Patanjali about the philosophy and practice of Yoga.

Z

- **Zen**: A school of meditation that began in Japan and China, inspired by the Sanskrit word dhyāna (ध्यान), which means deep focus or meditation. Zen teaches calmness, simplicity, and awareness—values that are very close to Yoga.

SURYA NAMASKAR
The Cyclic Greeting to the Sun

"Thank you, Sun, for giving us light and life."
- Uncle Vivek

Surya Namaskar (Sun Salutation) is an awesome cycle of 12 steps. It always begins and ends in the Prayer Pose, accompanied by a specific Mantra, showing that every journey starts with respect and returns with gratitude. Each movement flows into the next, stretching and energizing the whole body. What makes it special is that every step can be done with a mantra, saluting the Sun with twelve different names.

The 12 Steps with Mantras

1. Prayer Pose - नमस्कारासन (Namaskārāsana)

Stand tall, feet together. Join your palms at the heart. Focus your mind and begin with respect.

Mantra: ॐ ह्रां मित्राय नमः (Om Hrām Mitrāya Namah - Salutations to the friend of all).

2. Raised Arms Pose - हस्तोत्तानासन (Hastottānāsana)

Stretch both arms overhead and gently arch back, opening the chest. This wakes up your spine.

Mantra: ॐ ह्रीं रवये नमः (Om Hrīṃ Ravaye Namah - Salutations to the shining one).

3. Standing Forward Bend - पदहस्तासन (Padahastāsana)

Exhale and bend forward from the hips, placing hands near the feet. This stretches the back and legs.

Mantra: ॐ ह्रूं सर्या नमः (Om Hrum Sūryāya Namah - Salutations to the dispeller of darkness).

4. Equestrian Pose (Left Leg Back) - वाम अश्व सचंलनासन (Vāma Aśva Sanchalanāsana)

Step the left leg back, keep the right knee bent and look forward. This strengthens legs and opens hips.

Mantra: ॐ हैं भानवे नमः (Om Hraim Bhānave Namah - Salutations to the one who illumines).

5. Mountain Pose - पर्वतासन(Parvatāsana)

Press palms down, step back, and lift hips high to form an inverted "V." This builds core and arm strength.

Mantra: ॐ हौं खगाय नमः (Om Hraum Khagāya Namah - Salutations to the one who moves in the sky).

6. Salute with Eight Points - अष्टाङ्ग नमस्कार (Aṣṭāṅga Namaskāra)

Lower knees, chest, and chin to the floor while keeping hips raised. Eight parts of the body touch the ground. This builds resilience.

Mantra: ॐ हः पुष्णे नमः (Om Hrah Puṣṇe Namah - Salutations to the giver of strength).

7. Cobra Pose - भुजङ्गासन(Bhujangāsana)

Slide forward, lift chest, keep shoulders back and look up. This opens the chest and strengthens the spine.

Mantra: ॐ ह्रां हिरण्यगर्भाय नमः (Om Hrām Hiraṇyagarbhāya Namah - Salutations to the golden cosmic self).

8. Mountain Pose - पर्वतासन (Parvatāsana)

Lift hips again, return to the inverted "V." This stretches back, arms, and legs.

Mantra: ॐ ह्रीं मारिचये नमः (Om Hrīṃ Māricaye Namah - Salutations to the lord of rays).

9. **Equestrian Pose (Right Leg Forward)** - दक्षिण अश्व सचंलनासन(Dakṣiṇa Aśva Sanchalanāsana) Step the right leg forward, keep the left leg stretched back, look up. This balances both sides of the body.Mantra: ॐ ह्रीं आदित्याय नमः (Om Hrūm Ādityāya Namah - Salutations to the son of Aditi, the cosmic mother).

10. **Standing Forward Bend** - पदहस्तासन (Padahastāsana)
Bring both feet together and fold forward once again, stretching evenly.
Mantra: ॐ ह्रैं सवित्रे नमः (Om Hraim Savitre Namah - Salutations to the life-giver, the inspirer).

11. **Raised Arms Pose** - हस्तोत्तानासन (Hastottānāsana)
Sweep arms overhead and gently arch back. This fills the body with energy.
Mantra: ॐ ह्रौं अर्काय नमः (Om Hraum Arkāya Namah - Salutations to the one worthy of praise).

12. **Prayer Pose** - नमस्कारासन (Namaskārāsana)
Return palms together at the chest, calm and steady. You complete the cycle with gratitude.
Mantra: ॐ ह्रः भास्कराय नमः (Om Hrah Bhāskarāya Namah - Salutations to the source of light).

Original Mantra

Om Hrām Hrīm Hrūm Hraim Hraum Hrah - Mitra Ravi Sūrya Bhānu Khaga Puṣan Hiraṇyagarbha Marīci Āditya Savitṛ Arka Bhāskarebhyo Namo Namaha

पूर्ण मंत्र

ॐ ह्रां ह्रीं ह्रूं ह्रैं ह्रौं ह्रः । मित्र रवि सूर्य भानु खग पुष्ण् हिरण्यगर्भ मरीचि आदित्य सवितृ अर्क भास्करभ्यो नमो नमः ॥

Why It Is a Cycle

- Begins and ends with respect - shows wholeness.
- Every move + breath = full-body workout.
- Mantras remind us the Sun is not just a star, but a symbol of energy and life.

Takeaway

» Surya Namaskar = exercise + gratitude + energy.
» 12 simple poses flow smoothly.
» Mantras = honoring nature.

Alphabet Yoga

Go through the alphabet and name a yoga-related word for each letter. If you can't think of a word, feel free to create your own!
Example:

A-
B-
C-
D-
E-
F-
G-
H-
I-
J-

K-
L-
M-
N-
O-
P-
Q-
R-

S-
T-
U-
V-
W-
X-
Y-
Z-

YOGA CROSSWORD

Clues-

ACROSS

1. The process by which the body converts food into energy.
4. Hand gestures used in yoga and meditation to channel energy.
5. Concentration or focus, the sixth limb of Ashtanga Yoga.
6. Ethical rules in yoga about how we treat others and the world.
7. A sacred sound used for meditation.
9. 'Life energy' as per Chinese philosophy.

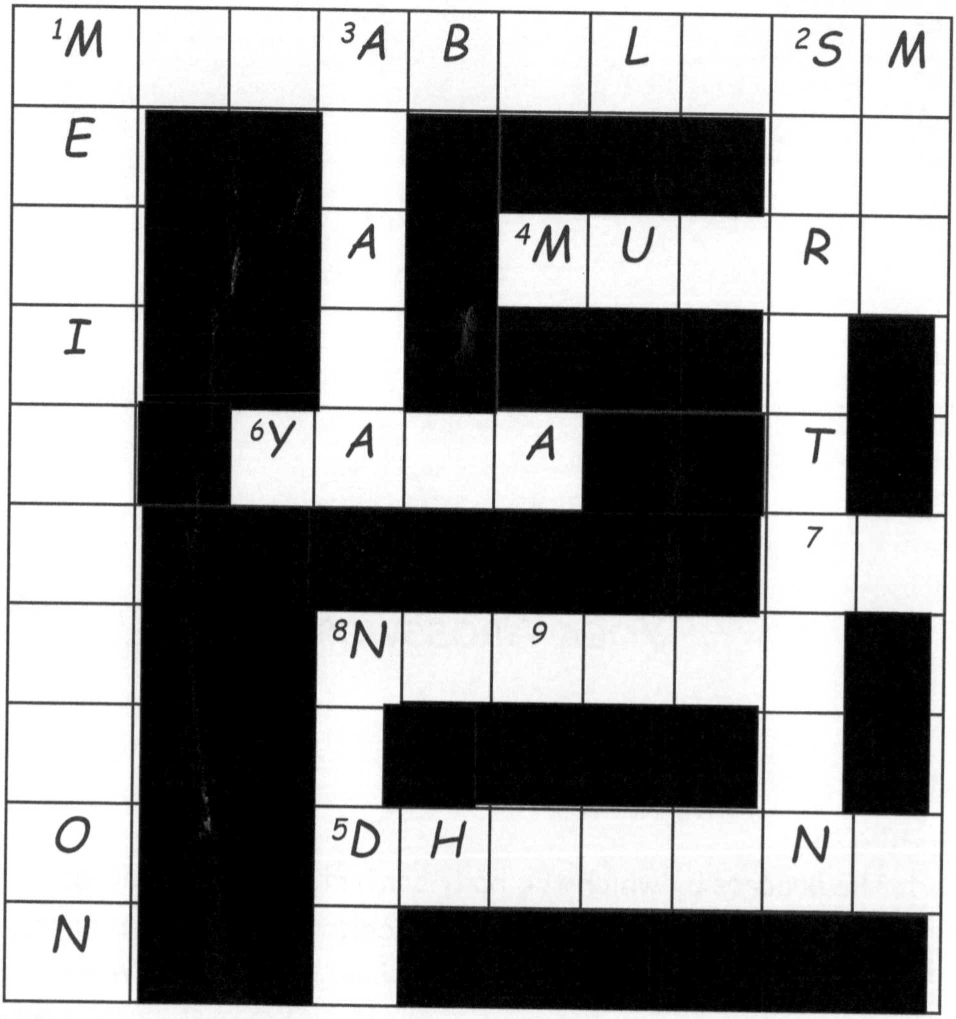

DOWN

1. A practice of focused stillness to calm the mind and improve awareness.
2. A brain chemical that helps regulate mood, sleep, and happiness.
3. A physical posture or pose practiced in yoga.
8. Energy channel through which Prana flows (main ones - Ida, Pingala, and Sushumna).

My Yoga Story!

Let your imagination run free as you write, draw, and color your own yoga story! [One-paged space provided]

Acknowledgements

This book grew with the curiosity, energy, and honesty of many young minds. To make it truly kid-friendly, we invited children to be part of the process — to read, question, suggest, and even challenge our ideas. Our special thanks to Arjun Hingorani, who worked with us as an associate throughout this journey. His enthusiasm, thoughtful suggestions, and cheerful presence helped shape the book in wonderful ways. Warm thanks to Sariva Tillu, whose thoughtful inputs, creative feedback, and sincere engagement brought depth and clarity to many ideas. Her youthful perspective helped make the content more lively, relatable, and interactive. Grateful appreciation to Pallavi Vyawahare, whose delightful illustrations and designs added colour, joy, and imagination, making this book visually engaging and appealing for readers of all ages.

We thank Subodh Tiwari, CEO of Kaivalyadhama for providing domain knowledge expertise. We thank Ms Mamta Bisht and Anjali Deshmukh, Yoga Teachers from Kaivalyadhama, for meticulous review and valuable comments to improve the accuracy and quality of content. We especially thank representatives of Gen Alpha and Gen Z generations for whom this book is meant — Chitra Godbole, Anshuman Gautam, Aradhya Kulkarni, Rihan Phansalkar, Tanvi Deshpande, Wishvaraj Puranik, and Sanchita Sangle — for their careful reading and frank feedback on early drafts. Their comments helped us see through a child's eyes and made the book more fun and friendly to read. We thank Dr Girish Tillu, Vaidya Sulakshana Bansode, Sumit Salunke, Prajakta Shinde for valuable comments. Our heartfelt gratitude to Ketaki and Tushar Hingorani, Mrs. Manisha and Dr. Vishnu Kulkarni, and Gayatri and Chaitanya Godbole, and Bhagyada Patwardhan for their constant encouragement, insights, and support.

A very special gratitude to Sunita Patwardhan, a Yoga teacher and mother of Bhushan Patwardhan, whose early guidance and inspiration laid the foundation for a lifelong journey.

We also extend our sincere thanks to Ashutosh Ramgir and his dedicated team at Sakal Publications for their professional support, enthusiasm, and commitment in bringing this book to life with such care and excellence. In addition, we thank all those who helped us in this journey through meaningful discussions, interactions, and engagements. Each of them, in their own way, contributed to making Yoga for Kids a book that speaks to children with joy, warmth, and wonder.

About the Creators

- **Bhushan Patwardhan** - Scientist, author, and educator known for bridging modern science with the wisdom and knowledge heritage of ancient Bharat. His work explores Ayurveda, Yoga, and integrative health, making complex ideas simple and relevant for young minds. His book Ayurveda for Kids is popular among readers of all ages.

- **Eeha Kulkarni** - Certified yoga instructor, healer, and engineer. Her scientific training deepens her Yogic practice, while her love for baking inspires mindfulness and precision. Having experienced the transformative power of Yoga through personal healing, she now shares it as a way of life and wellbeing.

- **Arjun Hingorani** - An energetic and imaginative Gen Alpha kid from the United States who loves reading, swimming, and fishing. His enthusiasm, curiosity, and creative ideas helped make the book more relatable for children everywhere.

- **Sariva Tillu** - A talented and thoughtful student of Microbiology with a keen interest in Ayurveda and Yoga. Her inquisitive mind, creativity, and passion added clarity, depth, and liveliness to the book, making it more engaging.

- **Pallavi Vyawahare** - An imaginative artist and designer whose illustrations and layouts brought life to every page. Her vibrant images and thoughtful visuals made this book attractive and engaging for children as well as readers of all ages.

About the Creation

Prof. Bhushan Patwardhan conceptualized this book, wrote the first draft, and undertook multiple revisions to shape its vision and message. Eeha Kulkarni refined, improved, and edited the manuscript to ensure accuracy and alignment with classical Yogic concepts. Together, they co-authored the book. Associate authors Arjun Hingorani and Sariva Tillu helped bring relevance to the children's world, adding freshness, curiosity, and an interactive spirit that connects well with Gen Alpha and Gen Z. Artist Pallavi Vyawahare enriched the book with her creative illustrations, design, and visual storytelling, making it appealing and joyful for young and grown-up readers alike. Together, the authors, associate authors, and artist created this unique book to introduce Yoga as a knowledge system for well-being—a bridge between timeless wisdom and the imagination of today's generation.

Write to us!

- Tried out a new Yoga pose?
- Performed an act of selflessness?
- Introduced your friends to yoga?
- Write to us with your photos!

Our Email: yoga4kidsbook@gmail.com

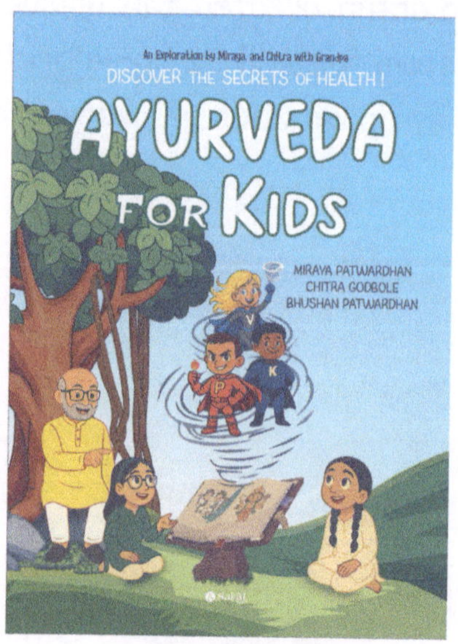